BEDTIME MEDITATIONS FOR KIDS

MEDITATION STORIES AND TALES FOR CHILDREN TO GO TO SLEEP.

AUTHOR

Sam Swift

Table of contents

THE INTRODUCTION TO BEDTIME STORY **5**

- The Bedtime Story and Reason for Reading One Each Night 5
- Best Bedtime Meditations for Kids 5
- The most effective method to best guide your child to ponder 8
- For what reason is Bedtime Stories Important for Children 10

BEDTIME STORIES FOR CHILDREN **14**

THE SEA ANIMAL PROTAGONIST STORIES **14**

- 1. The Starfish – Every Small Bit Matters 14
- 2. The Dolphin and the Shark 15
- 3. The Little Fish in the Big Ocean 16
- 4. Bintu the Whale 17
- 5. The Undersea Adventure of the Blue Diamond 18
- 6. The Lucky Octopus 20
- 7. Good Morning Fish 22
- 8. The fish who could peruse 25
- 9. The City Under The Sea 27
- 10.The Witch took from a little 33
- 11.The Princess and the Prince cried out a voice. 35
- 12. PHILIP, THE SEA WOLF 40
- 13. The Rainbow Fish Story 41
- 14. The desolate starfish 42
- 15. The Dinosaur Camping 46
- 16. The Unhappy Big Fish 47
- 17. The Tale Of Three Fishes 48

10 JUNGLE ANIMALS PROTAGONIST STORIES FOR CHILDREN BEDTIME **51**

- What Is A Jungle Bedtime Story? 51
- Create Memories Together 51
- Benefits Of Bedtime Stories 51
- 1. Baby Bubba goes to the Jungle 53
- 2. Monster in the Jungle 56

- 2. A Dance in the Forest with the Parrot 56
- 3. The Clever Monkey 59
- 4. The Wolf And The Seven Young Goslings 60
- 5. A Life in the Woods 62
- 6. A Caterpillar's Voice 68
- 7. The Mouse That Roared Story 70
- 8. Crocodile and Monkey Story 70
- 9. The Bowman And The Lion 71
- 10.THE LITTLE JACKALS AND THE LION 72
- 11.THE COUNTRY MOUSE AND THE CITY MOUSE 74
- 12.LITTLE JACK ROLL AROUND 75
- 13. The Last Dinosaurs 77
- 14. The Mocking Tiger 78
- 15. Manute the Brave 78
- 16. The Mysterious Juggling Clown 79
- 17. A Day With The Pigs 80
- 18. A Ray of Moonlight 81
- 19. Never Make Fun of a Rhino 81
- 20. The Frog King Fairy Tale Story 82
- 21. A Wish For Christmas 85
- 22. A Perfect Christmas 87

OTHER BEDTIME STORIES 92

- 1. A Seaside Adventure (Ears Mouse) 92
- 2. The Swans and the Turtle 96
- 3. The Three Little Pigs 97
- 4. The Cat and The Mouse in Partnership 100
- 5. Tropical Adventure in the Magic Shed 102
- 6. The Adventures of Sprinkles The Cat; The King 103
- 7. A Queer Friendship 105
- 8. Dinosaurs In My Bed 106
- 9. Ginger and the six felines 109
- 10. Kyle the Monkey 111

THE INTRODUCTION TO BEDTIME STORY

The Bedtime Story and Reason for Reading One Each Night

Perusing bedtime stories, fairy tales, and society tales with your child before bed is a family custom of storytelling that has been around for many years. Offering a bedtime story to your children is storytelling in its most perfect structure. It's a chance not simply to share a straightforward bedtime story to be overlooked, yet spending on a lifetime of exercises from the individuals who preceded us. It's a chance to associate with your child every night.

Perusing famous bedtime stories, for example, the cherished tales of Cinderella, Rapunzel, Pinocchio, Snow White, and more assistance slide a child into sleep. Perusing bedtime stories every night to your child has been demonstrated the best method to improve perusing and jargon aptitudes. Our stories likewise show virtues, for example, generosity, companionship, and sympathy. Peruse a bedtime story and offer in the enchantment of storytelling with your child today around evening time!

Offer our bedtime stories and great fairy tales in a daily custom of learning. While a bedtime story may be viewed as something to hurry through so as to get to the snappiest decision, a genuinely necessary rest for a bustling child, it very well may be the most enchanting snapshot of the day. Taking that child to a universe of discovery through a story will, without a doubt, leave an enduring impression. Make the most of our unique assortment of stories that have been kid-tried and contain positive good messages and qualities.

Best Bedtime Meditations for Kids

What does the word 'Bed-time' evoke for you? Pictures of cushioned pads and fresh white sheets? In case you're the parent of a young child, odds are the pictures in your mind are not exactly so quiet!
Bedtime is frequently the most testing piece of the day, particularly for the children.
Ever had a go at putting a child to bed? It's the hardest activity on the planet! In any case, acquaint your children with meditation, and you will assist them with sleeping better, and be balanced people tomorrow.

Sleep inconvenience isn't a thing of simply the adults. Children can confront sleeping difficulties, particularly during little child years, when you are too eager even to consider exploring their general surroundings. Bedtime can transform into a combat zone when these little people don't comply with the clock. There are many attempted and tried methods that appear to work in such circumstances. These incorporate setting an individualized bedtime schedule, setting a wake-up time, making a predictable bedtime routine, and turning contraptions and TVs off at any rate 2 hours before bedtime. It likewise enables when you to make a sleep instigating condition by perusing bedtime stories, dodging exercises, and games that cause them to be too energized and confining nourishments that contain caffeine and sugar. What's more, there are numerous meditation methods that appear to help in putting your little one to sleep.

Meditation and children? It sounds like something that is alongside difficult to accomplish, yet given our hyper-tactile condition and unnecessary stimulation as the day progressed, most children discover it incredibly extreme to slow down for the evening. With these meditations for children, you can enable your children to remain zen before they sleep around evening time.

For 3-6-year-olds

This is the age when children think that its difficult to sit still, not to mention center and loosen up following a bustling day. In the event that you have a child in this age gathering, you have to assist them with settling on the cognizant choice to start turning off and relaxing, as bedtime draws nearer. Attempt to get them to discuss their feelings, what's occurred as the day progressed, and help them de-stress at their level. A book or two, and some peaceful time (between 45 seconds and 2 minutes), likewise fills in as children's meditation and keeps them grounded.

Over 6 Years

Continuously recall that stillness isn't an idea that comes simple to children, and as a parent, you have to assist them with accomplishing that objective of all-out relaxation. With children over 6, this can be accomplished through a few methods. For instance, you can make light of a snappy breeze game with them. Make them rests with their eyes shut and afterward starting from the toes, stir your way up as it's been said goodnight to each body part. Sometimes, giving them an article or a delicate toy to clutch additionally encourages them to get into a relaxed, thoughtful edge that is basic at this hour.

The intensity of the music

Music has the ability to calm one into a daze, and help with relaxation. You can seat your child, or make them rests, and afterward play some relieving music to them. The other method to do this is by getting them to murmur a tune or sing a melody in their minds while contacting the tips of every one of their fingers all the while. This will assist them with centering and ponder. Children of any age can do this.

Taking full breaths

This may appear to be more earnestly than it is. Children also need to, at some stage, become mindful of the intensity of breathing right. Get them to tune in to their own breathing, check their breaths, and attempt and progressively take longer breaths. Not at all like uplifted mindfulness about a procedure that is regular and fundamental, yet answerable for soothing a ton of their anxiety and squirming.

Children are experiencing childhood in an alternate time age. The advanced age is such a lot faster and stronger than what we needed to adapt to when we were kids.

Presently like never before, children are assaulted with impressions, messages, desires which, when combined with the losses of current living, over-booking, and long school days, can significantly impact on their psychological prosperity. Also, today tragically more children than any time in recent memory endure with stress, wretchedness, anxiety, and misery.

One hour less sleep.

Sleep, or rather its absence, is one of the principal signs for guardians that something may be topsy turvy.

Much the same as grown-ups – or possibly more – children are similarly as powerless to the entanglements of a stressful day, and increasingly more falsehood conscious around evening time, unfit to 'switch off' and with dashing considerations. Stress is frequently an overriding element, and many make some hard memories giving up.

As a rule, children today sleep one hour short of what we completed 25 years prior. Like grown-ups, sleep issues in children will, in general, have a thump on impact, regularly showing in crabbiness and absence of center at school. What's more, having a child who can't nod off is additionally debilitating for guardians.

Why children can't sleep.

The world we show our children are turning such a great amount of faster than the one our folks indicated us. It is said that a child today gets as a lot of boost in one day, as their distant grandparents did in a whole year when they were children. Obviously, this is speculation, yet consider it for a minute.
The ideal approach to show our children how to explore is to make sure to explore ourselves. The human race isn't intended for progressing exercises. We are intended to utilize vitality, and afterward, rest to refuel. Yet, we appear to have disregarded the resting part. Barely astounding, then that such a large number of guardians additionally experience difficulty sleeping.

We have to outfit our children with these assets to empower them to manage all that society needs to toss at them, the steady overload of data and messages, and to assist them with recharging.
We can't stop advancement, and we can't change society overnight. What we can do, however, is show our children how to explore in the hurried world they are growing up in. Children truly need their sleep, and we can instruct them methods to quiet down and see the harmony required as ready to give up.

How meditation can help.
As various as children seem to be, pretty much every child savors the experience of hearing adoration and heart vitality, which numerous meditations offer. Learning how to turn up their self-esteem can give children so much solace that they relax and nod off.

A recorded guided meditation can be a decent spot to start in the event that you are not yourself acquainted with meditation. In any case, I prescribe that you generally sit with your child and tune in along in the event that you choose to play a meditation for your child. Your essence is very important. Too regularly, I hear that guardians leave the space to go fix something different, while the child is tuning in to meditation. The result of the meditation on the off chance that you remain and rests with your child and relax is so much better. In the event that your more established child demands that you leave the room, that would be alright, yet a younger child would probably need you to remain.

The most effective method to best guide your child to ponder.

Far superior is perusing a meditation to your child yourself. Request a book with child meditations or go to your library. At the point when you read the meditation to your child, your vitality helps the child a great deal, and your direction makes your child have a sense of security. To your child, no voice is better than yours, on the grounds that it joins all that you are and all that you transmit.

If you choose to peruse a meditation to your child at bedtime, getting mindful of your vitality as a parent is significant. Perusing meditations when you can be available, adoring, and quiet at bedtime can assist your child in finding internal harmony, cherish, and even self-esteem. Here's the manner by which to do that:

1. Pick a time when you feel better, and have the vitality to enable your child to manage another method of nodding off.

2. Turn off the screens before bedtime, including your own.

3. Slow down the most recent hour before perusing.

4. Let your child take a warm, relaxing shower. Far and away superior – end the shower with a delicate back rub with a decent oil.

5. Stay quiet and cherishing in your vitality regardless of whether your child experiences issues with the new method. Your vitality, state of mind, and method for speaking with your child profoundly influence how rapidly he/she quiets down. You can peruse even start by perusing one of your child's preferred books, so the new meditation book turns into an extra.

6. Lay down alongside your child and show him/her, you have the opportunity to peruse the book in a quiet and comfortable manner. Cuddle up. Furthermore, in the event that you nod off yourself, that may be exactly what you need.

7. Stay quiet, cherishing regardless of whether your child wouldn't like to close his eyes or moves around. At the point when children start to inhale and move their thoughtfulness regarding their body, which many guided meditations will show them, it is normal that they need to move around a piece. For certain children shutting their eyes can be somewhat of a test. Simply request that they stare at a particular spot in the room until they are prepared to close their eyes. Welcome them tenderly into the meditation.
8. Speak in a quiet, cherishing voice and make sure to make stops.

9. In the days after the meditation, you can converse with your child about the experience. Tune in to your child – there is a long way to go.

10. Encourage your child to draw – or expound on the pictures or sentiments he/she sees or encounters during meditation.

Appreciate the ride while pondering with your child. Numerous children have a lot of simpler time thinking to their souls than grown-ups. What's more, from multiple points of view, children can assist guardians with turning up the affection for themselves also.

At the point when a child reflects, they enter the Relaxation Response, and their body can approach doing what it normally does, processing, fixing, etc. At the point when a child is vexed, hyper upset, on edge, furious, and so on.
This alarm state is vital for loads of various reasons, specifically endurance, anyway it is additionally important that the child returns to the Relaxation Response with the goal that they are quiet, have a sense of security, and can tune in and learn.
At the point when a child learns to think, they not just enter the Relaxation Response all the more routinely, they additionally become increasingly present, mindful, and can self-manage. They become progressively mindful of what they are doing, how they are responding, and that they have a decision. It improves their mindfulness, and they become more acquainted with their emotions, which will have expansive impacts well into adulthood. Mindfulness, at that point, makes drive control and advances the conduct of reacting as opposed to responding.
These meditations can manage you and your child to mysterious and awesome spots, to places inside that, are sheltered and quiet, and back with a bunch of issues. If it's not too much trouble recall, nonetheless, that while meditation offers an awesome help, it doesn't supplant professional restorative or mental counsel. Meditation can be utilized connected at the hip with whatever treatment or counsel you might be following.

Offering Guided Meditation to children offers them a chance to encounter a spot inside that is sheltered, a spot where they can come to feel love, self-esteem, delight, joy, and all the charming sentiments we appreciate feeling — a position of stillness and harmony. You will see a moving change in your child when they consistently contemplate and maybe need to go to that spot as well!

For what reason is Bedtime Stories Important for Children

As a parent, your prime concern is your child's wellbeing and prosperity. Wellbeing is dealt with when you give nutritious nourishment, and a sound and safe condition for your child will deal with their prosperity. Alongside these, guardians need their children to grow up to be a decent individual throughout everyday life.

Numerous guardians are in the propensity for perusing or imparting bedtime stories to their children. They, for the most part, accept it as fun action. The main thing that most guardians need to understand that sharing or describing bedtime stories can be instrumental in building your child's character also.

Investing energy during bedtime story sessions additionally have some different benefits that are referenced beneath:

- Quality time – Reading or describing stories assist guardians with investing some quality energy with children before they end their day. A ton of sharing occurs during that time.

- Strengthens the family bond – After a long chaotic day where children are occupied with school, play, TV, and guardians are caught up with taking care of family unit errands and professional duties, bedtime story session allows guardians and children to fortify their relations and bond with one another.

- Relaxes the brain – Bedtime stories are an incredible method for relaxing a child's psyche. The disposition is set for an agreeable and sound sleep as children snuggle up in bed.

- Enhances creative mind – Many of the storybooks have fairy tales, stories of superheroes, some antiquated characters, animals, forests, and experiences that trigger the creative mind of young ones on the grounds that such scenes are not regular in their everyday lives.

- Creative reasoning and critical thinking abilities – Bedtime story sessions can turn into an extraordinary instrument in creating innovative intuition for children too. Guardians can generally peruse or describe stories with fascinating turns. Respite before the end and request that the child proposes a conclusion to the story, or you may portray a couple of lines and afterward request that the child proceed. It will be fun and will assist the child with thinking inventively just as glance out answers for the conceivable issue circumstances.

- Improves relational abilities – During these story sessions, guardians and children get an opportunity to associate and examine the characters and the storyline. Numerous new words are perused and talked about — this outcome in improved relational abilities and upgraded jargon.

Kaitlin concedes that bedtime stories give her those couple of seconds when her girl shares her desires, creative mind, and her fantasies. She likewise shares episodes from her everyday existence with her mom. It causes Kaitlin to keep in contact with what is happening in her 8-year-old girl's life.

- Increases capacity to focus – Most children appreciate tuning in to stories as they discover them fascinating. It can likewise be made intriguing by describing it with the assistance of outward appearances and hand developments. Tuning in and perusing bedtime stories in a routine can improve the capacity to focus and listening to the abilities of children.

- Source of motivation – Most of these stories for children have a decent good toward the end, and they can be useful in teaching fundamental abilities like genuineness, fearlessness, regard, liberality, and so forth. Such stories additionally have moving biographies or circumstances that can propel the child to be an effective and great individual..

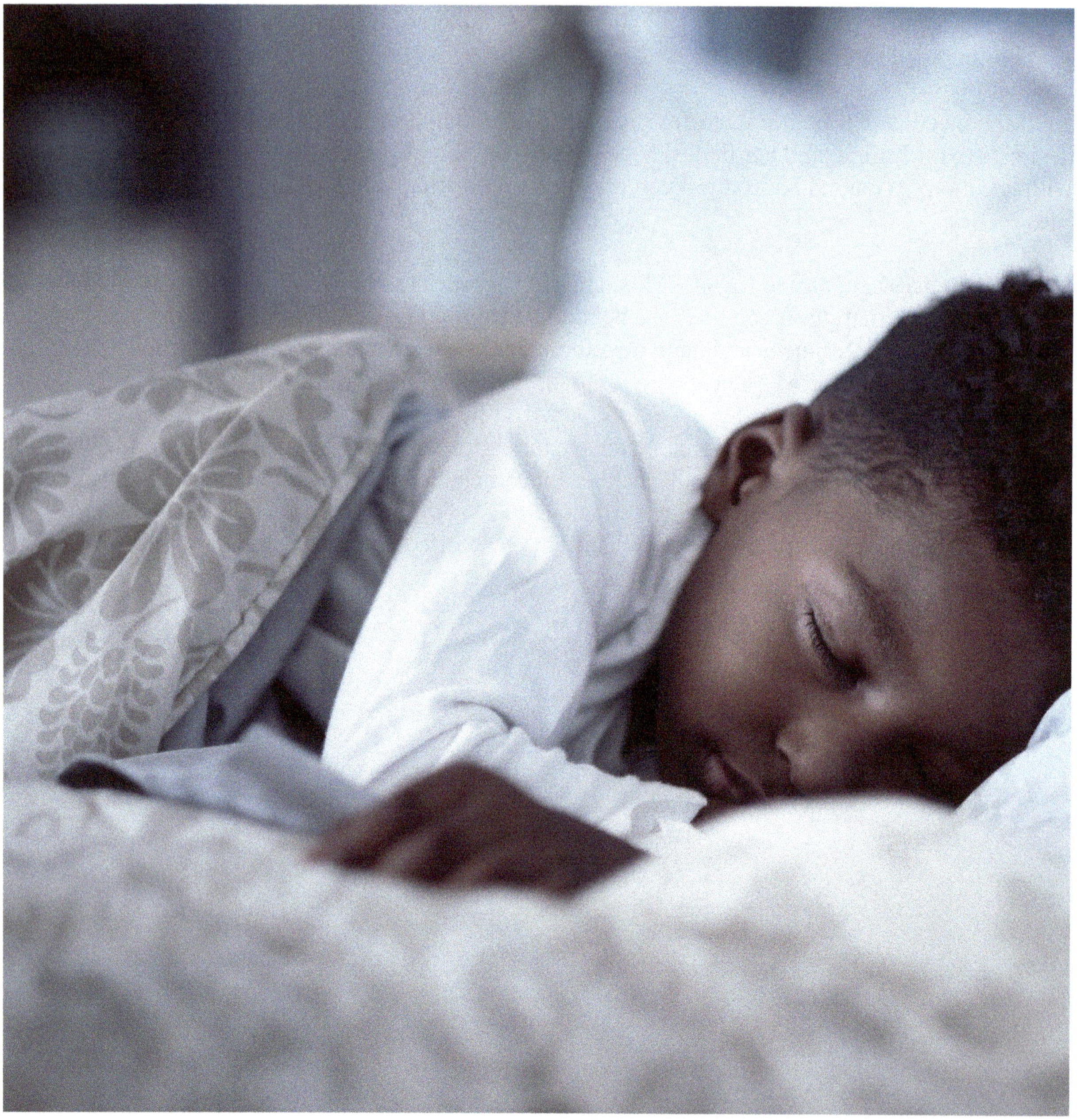

BEDTIME STORIES FOR CHILDREN

THE SEA ANIMAL PROTAGONIST STORIES

1. The Starfish – Every Small Bit Matters

Some time ago, there was an elderly person who used to go to the sea each morning. He would initially go for a comfortable walk along the seashore, and afterward would plunk down to do his composition.

One night, there was a loathsome tempest. The enormous tempest had passed, and the elderly person strolled down to the seashore. He found the tremendous seashore covered with starfish. They extended the extent that the eye could see, every which way.

Far out there, the elderly person saw a little kid strolling towards him. Be that as it may, the kid was not strolling straightforwardly towards him. Rather he would stop now and again, twist down as though to get something from the sand. At that point, he would fix up and toss something out of sight of the sea.

As he developed nearer, the elderly person got out, "Hello! May I ask, would it be that you are tossing into the sea?"

The young kid strolled fixed and approached the elderly person with a starfish in his grasp. He answered, "I am tossing the starfish once more into the sea. The tempest cleaned them up on to the seashore the previous evening. Presently the tide is out of sight, and the starfish can't come back to the sea without anyone else. At the point when the sun gets excessively high, they will kick the bucket as a result of the warmth. So I am tossing them once more into the water before that occurs."

The elderly person was befuddled and thought about whether the kid was essentially moronic. He would not any way like to sound discourteous. "Be that as it may, there must be a huge number of starfish on this seashore. It is difficult to spare every one of them. I'm apprehensive you won't have the option to make a big deal about a distinction", he said.

The kid twisted down, got another starfish, and tossed it to the extent he could into the water. At that point, he turned and grinned at the elderly person, and stated, "I spared one more starfish. It made a distinction to that one!"

2. The Dolphin and the Shark

Once upon a time, there was a shark named Jaz and a dolphin named Steve. They lived in the sea, not very a long way from an excellent sandy seashore, a tall beacon, and a dull, dim bog.

Presently Jaz and Steve knew one another. However, they weren't the best of companions! Steve is blessed with two sisters, and they all played together and dealt with one another, and were cheerful in the cool blue water.

As it is, Jaz swam alone, he had no siblings or sisters, and nobody to play with, and that made him exceptionally crotchety. Thus he went through his days swimming languidly, feeling frustrated about himself, and simply being mean.

Jaz's preferred thing was to assault Steve and his sisters. He would make a plunge the water, sneaking close to the base, and afterward, when he saw the dolphins playing close to the surface, he would swim as hard as he could toward them and attempt to chomp their tails! In any case, the dolphins consistently observed him coming, and they would come up out of the water and remain on their tails, and whistle and snicker, the manner in which dolphins do, and they generally figured out how to keep simply far from Jazs huge sharp teeth.

I don't think Jaz truly needed to get them isn't that right? In such a case that he got them and ate them, well... he wouldn't have some good times any longer. In any case, you never think about sharks, so Steve and his sisters were consistently vigilant for Jaz the mope.

At some point, while Steve was swimming independent from anyone else, and Jaz was pursuing him, they got exceptionally near the shore. Steve jumped out of the water with Jaz directly behind him, and the two of them saw something exceptionally bizarre on the seashore. There, driving out of the bog, were unusual tracks in the sand! Steve quit swimming, and Jaz quit pursuing, and they skimmed and pondered about the surprising impressions before them.

They had never observed imprints that way! "I wonder on the off chance that it was a duck charged platypuses?" said Steve. "I don't think so," answered Jaz, "I'll wager it was a Red-Breasted Hairy Headed Knee, Walker!"

In any case, since neither of those animals was found in those parts all the time, they continued pondering. They thought possibly it had been a Big Bellied Widget Gobbler, or a Black and White Thingy, or maybe a Hooty Snooty Crawler. Be that as it may, they simply didn't know what had made those amusing, enormous impressions!

Out of the blue, they heard something coming, something was rearranging along the seashore. They could nearly observe it now, it was drawing nearer and closer, and afterward, there it was! It was much more interesting than anything they had suspected of! There, coming at them, getting ever closer was.........

....a by golly incredible enormous green gator, wearing an interesting cap and raggedy overalls! Furthermore, he was moving!

Indeed, they thought this was the most amusing sight they had ever observed, yet at that point, they heard music as well! Also, the music was getting stronger and stronger, and out of the sides of their eyes, they saw...oh, it just couldn't be!

There, leaving the marsh, was a frog playing the banjo! Furthermore, over there, strolling towards them up the seashore, was a raccoon playing a fiddle! Also, soon the three peculiar animals were directly before Jaz and Steve, and the incredible green gator moved, and they were all making some awesome memories!

Jaz and Steve were surprised and dumbfounded, and they just skimmed and watched and tuned in as the croc moved to tune after tune. What's more, Steve applauded his flippers, and Jaz acclaimed with his balances, and they thought they had never had a ton of fun.

The music and moving endured throughout the evening, and the sun was starting to set when the two performers and the artist started to head out in their own direction. The frog returned to the marsh, the raccoon jogged off down the seashore, and the gator went into the stones close to the beacon.
What's more, as they watched, they suspected what they had seen.
Jaz had been pondering what had occurred. He had seen three altogether different animals getting along well, and being the best of companions. He had perceived how glad they were as one. What's more, he had seen himself coasting next to each other with a dolphin, them two getting a charge out of similar music and moving.
Jaz contemplated how forlorn his life was, swimming in solitude, without any companions, and being surly. He had thought extremely hard about these things. Thus, he chose what he should do, and he turned gradually toward the dolphin and swam gradually up to him and started to mention to him what he thought.
The sun was splendid yellow as it came up out of the sea the following morning, and the sky was a lovely shade of blue. Furthermore, in the event that somebody had been remaining on the shore, watching out over the water, they would have seen four balances slicing through the tides and waves. The three dolphins and a shark, yet the shark wasn't chasing Steve and his sisters, he was playing with them! Jaz had revealed to Steve how tired he was of being desolate and testy. He revealed to him how severely he needed a few companions. Also, he disclosed to him how brilliant it had been to see the frog, and the raccoon, and the gator, playing and moving and being the best of companions. Furthermore, Jaz felt that if three animals as various as those could do it, well, he and the dolphins could as well.
Presently they all swam together, and played together, and dealt with each other, and were extremely upbeat. What's more, every so often, when the sun and the mists and the sea were perfect, they would be sufficiently fortunate to get a look at the frog, and the raccoon, and the extraordinary green croc playing and moving in the sand.

3. The Little Fish in the Big Ocean

Once upon a time in the olden days, there lived a fish called George. George lived in the water, as all fish do; however, something was distinctive about George, he didn't care for the water. He he would discover something that he didn't care for. To start with, he said that the stones were too enormous. At that point, he said that the stones were excessively little. Nothing would please him together with the other fish in his school, all fish have a place with a school, would attempt to perk him up. They didn't comprehend why he was despondent. They adored swimming around in the shallow water and being as one.

The school lived in the waterfront waters of South Florida. This water was loaded with life and warmth. There was, in every case, a lot of nourishment and movement, and there were always exciting things happening for these fish. In any case, for reasons unknown, George felt anxious and discontent, and he needed more. At some point, a major, old, and insightful fish came to visit his school. He listened eagerly. The old and shrewd one was recounting huge waters and boundless swimming. He was recounting incredible whales and enormous fish. He was additionally telling about incredible light and haziness. Abruptly George needed to encounter this as well. The other fish in the school were not intrigued, yet George was excited. He swam with the large fish towards these tremendous waters with incredible dreams.

Before long, the water started to feel cold, and he saw monster fish that looked extremely ravenous. He would have been apprehensive about his life. However, he was excessively energized by the new sights. Before long, they went to a cavern, and they found a protected spot for the night with nourishment close by.

George loved it in the cavern. It was extremely peaceful, and he could hear quiet sounds. The musical sound appeared to be originating from a long separation. In any event, when the huge fish swam away, George chose to remain. This was against all typical fish impulses, as fish needs to be with other fish. Nonetheless, as I said prior, George was not a typical fish. The resonant sound interested him, and he couldn't quit tuning in to it. He even started to recognize the various tones and sorts of sound. He tuned in, and he tuned in. He didn't eat or move since he was so bustling tuning in. The more he tuned in, the more he started to comprehend who he truly was. The more he tuned in, the more he fell into alternate mindfulness, and soon he overlooked that he was a fish and that he didn't care for the water.

One day the enormous and savvy fish was swimming by the cavern, and he considered George, so he went into the cavern. There he discovered George exactly where he had left him a long while back. George had changed nonetheless and didn't appear to be identical by any means. He was sparkling in an extraordinary manner, and his breathing was incredibly moderate. George perceived the old and astute fish and invited him.
George was presently additionally old and insightful, and the two remaining the cavern together.

4. Bintu the Whale

Bintu, the Whale, was huge - enormous -, and desolate - forlorn. For a particular time, she had needed nothing to do with anybody, and she had gotten more troubled and more troubled. At whatever point anybody attempted to draw near to her and cheer her up, Bintu would get off.
Many ideas that she was the most disagreeable whale on the planet, and they started disregarding her. They did as such, regardless of the way that old Turga, a multi-year-old sea turtle, disclosed to them that Bintu had consistently been a decent, kind whale.

At some point, Dido, a young dolphin, heard the entire story and chose to pursue the whale covertly. She discovered that Bintu carried on abnormally. The whale would beat her mouth against the stones, jeopardize herself by swimming between the greatest waves and the coast, and go to the seafloor and eat sand. Nobody knew it, yet Bintu had frightfully terrible breath in light of the fact that a little fish had got caught in an edge of her mouth. This issue humiliated Bintu so much that she didn't set out to address anybody. At the point when Dido understood this, she offered to help. However, Bintu would not like to trouble her with her awful breath. Nor did she need anybody to discover.
"I don't need them to think I have awful breath," said Bintu.
"Is that why you've invested so a lot of energy away from everybody?" addressed Dido, incapable of trusting it. "They don't think you have awful breath, they believe you're upsetting, exhausting, and dissatisfied, and that you despise everybody. Do you feel that is better?"

Bintu understood that her pride - she overstated modesty, and not allowing anybody to help - had made a considerably more noteworthy issue. Loaded with lament, she solicited Dido to expel the remaining parts from the fish in her mouth.

At the point when this was done, Bintu started addressing everybody once more. Be that as it may, she needed to endeavor to be acknowledged again by her companions. Bintu concluded that never again would she neglect to request help when she truly required it.

5. The Undersea Adventure of the Blue Diamond

There was a mermaid, a crab, a sea-lion, a sea-horse, and a sea turtle. They all lived respectively in the Great Pacific Ocean. One day as they were taking a pleasant virus swim, they ran over a guide to a money box. On it was denoted the Great Castle of Gold (GCG). There were no headings! So every one of the companions set off to locate the Great Castle of Gold, arranged for a long swim in the sea.

They swam for two days with no karma. On the third day, as they were swimming, they met a fish named Tory. She was lost and didn't have the foggiest idea about the way home.

"Hello, can you all assist me with returning home?" Tory inquired.

"Gee, golly. We can't," they answered.

"Come go along with us! We are going for a long swim to discover a fortune." Said the mermaid.

"Goodness! I saw something shining on my way!" said Tory.

"Where did you see it?" yelled everybody, enthusiastically.

"It was entirely far away." Said Tory. "Be that as it may, I think I recall! I recollect! I recall!" And she started swimming ceaselessly.

Everybody pursued Tory energetically. In the wake of swimming for 60 minutes, they arrived at the Great Castle of Gold.

"Presently, we have to discover the chest." Said the mermaid.

Gracious! I know. We should thump on the Castle entryway." Said Tory.

So they all thumped on the entryway and paused.

Before long, somebody opened the mansion entryway. It was the blue witch. The blue witch was a decent witch. She was benevolent and supportive, and excellent. She had a silver and jewel tiara. Every one of the companions was astonished to see such a wonderful witch. They thought all witches were terrible.

"Hello there. We are the sea animals of the Great Pacific Ocean. We found a guide to a money box in the Great Castle of Gold and came here searching for it." Said the mermaid.

"Welcome to the Great Castle of Gold." Said the Blue Witch. "I am the gatekeeper of this royal residence. I can let you take the money box. In any case, before that, you will all need to finish a test."

The sea animals were all exceptionally glad to hear that. In any case, they were likewise stressed over what the test would be.

"Ooh! I love difficulties!" said Tory.

The Blue Witch grinned and stated, "In the manor garden, there is an exceptionally overwhelming Blue Diamond, which is watched by an old mermaid. Legend says that whoever can get the Blue Diamond and set it back into the Great Castle of Gold can take the money box. In the event that all of you can do that, I will let you take the money box."

The mermaid, crab, sea-lion, sea-pony, and sea turtle set off towards the mansion garden. There they saw a huge precious stone. An old mermaid was sleeping beside it.

The sea-lion approached the old mermaid and stated, "Hi. We are here to attempt to bring the precious blue stone into the palace. May we?"

The old mermaid woke up and stated, "Yes, sure. I have never observed any individual who could lift it! You may attempt in the event that you need to."

All the five companions took a stab at getting the precious stone. Be that as it may, not one of them could move it an inch. At that point, Tory ventured up to attempt. The companions took a gander at her and said confusedly, "Ca-would you be able to get it?"

Tory stated, "I'll attempt!" And, gracious happiness! She had the option to lift the precious stone with one hand! Everybody stared at her in wonder.

"Hello, fellas, where do you need me to take this enormous bit of bluestone to?" asked Tory.

"Into the palace," said everybody together.

They all strolled into the palace with the blue witch driving them. Inside the château, they set the blue jewel inside McFee, the mystical well.

The blue witch went to the companions and Tory and stated, "Congrats, you can take the money box. Be that as it may since Tory was the person who got the Blue Diamond, you should ensure that she turns into a piece of your gathering as well."

At that point, she went to Tory and stated, "I will give her a mystical house. At whatever point you head off to someplace and lose your direction, you simply need to state, 'Abra-ca-dabra, zippetty-Zapp. Where is my home, come to me fast.' And your home will show up before you. So you will never be lost again."

All six companions were currently extremely upbeat. They took the money box and the guide and started swimming back home where they all lived respectively cheerfully until the end of time.

6. The Lucky Octopus

A children's short story with jargon and appreciation practices for young learners of English. With sound. Composed and read by Tara Benwell. Level: lower-middle of the road

Ollie, the octopus, just had seven legs.

"The last one will develop," the sea specialist said the day Ollie was conceived.

"In any case, when?" asked Ollie's mom. She was exceptionally pitiful.

"When Ollie turns eight years old," the specialist said.

For seven years, Ollie's siblings and sisters prodded her about her missing leg. She was the youngest octopus in the family. Her sister Olivia was the most established.

"Ollie just has seven legs since she isn't a piece of our genuine family," Olivia told the other sea animals one day.

It was an untruth, yet everybody trusted Olivia on the grounds that she was the most established.

At the point when the other sea animals messed around like tag and found the stowaway, Ollie's sibling Oscar wouldn't let Ollie play.

"You can't get a fish with just seven legs," Oscar said. "Proceed to discover a companion that has an additional leg to play with."

Ollie searched around the sea, yet there weren't any caring sea animals to play with. She was desolate.

One day Ollie's sibling Orlando saw Ollie playing independent from anyone else in the seaweed. He was extremely glad.

"Think about what I discovered today, Ollie!" Orlando said. "A money box. It is from a ship, and it is brimming with delightful gems."

"Would I be able to see it?" Ollie inquired. "I have constantly longed for seeing a money box."

"I'm not demonstrating it to anybody!" Orlando said. "Particularly not a little octopus with just seven legs."

Ollie returned home and disclosed to her mom that she was miserable. "Everybody treats me diversely in light of the fact that I just have seven legs," she said.

"Try not to stress," her mom said. "Tomorrow is your eighth birthday celebration, and you will at long last develop another leg! At that point, you will never be desolate."

That night Ollie envisioned that she developed another leg. Everybody celebrated and ate flavorful nourishment. She was so upbeat. Yet, the following day, when Ollie woke up and checked her legs, there were still just seven.

Ollie stowed away in the seaweed fix and cried. She was so dismal. Abruptly a sea fairy showed up. It was the littlest animal Ollie had ever observed.

"You are the fortunate octopus I have been hanging tight for," the sea fairy said.

"I am?" Ollie said.

"Truly. Just the most fortunate octopus gets the opportunity to make three wishes."

Ollie knew precisely what to want.

"First, I wish that Olivia was straightforward," Ollie said.

"Your desire is allowed. Presently you have two additional desires," the fairy said.

"Second, I wish that Oscar was caring."

"What's more, presently he is," the fairy said. "Furthermore, what is your last wish?"

"Finally, I wish that Orlando was reasonable," Ollie said.

Before the minor sea fairy vanished, she disclosed to Ollie that she was the kindest octopus in the entire sea. "I wish that the entirety of your birthday blessings from heaven," the sea fairy said before she swam away.

When Ollie returned home, her family was sitting tight for her. "Shock!" they said at the same time.

"I got you a present," Oscar said. "It's a lovely pearl accessory!"

"Much thanks to you," Ollie said. "You are benevolent."

"I prepared a tasty cake for you," Orlando said. "What's more, I welcomed the entirety of the sea animals to impart it to us."

"You are exceptionally reasonable," Ollie said. "Much obliged to you for sharing."

"I'm exceptionally grieved, I don't have a present for you," Olivia said. "I overlooked it was your birthday."

"That is alright," Ollie said. "You are straightforward. Much obliged to you."

Ollie's mom swam over to her little girl with a red birthday expand.

"I'm so cheerful for you, Ollie," she said.

"Why, Mother?"

"See, you've at last developed your eighth leg!" Ollie's mom attached the inflatable to her girl's new leg.

It was the most joyful day of Ollie's life.

7. Good Morning Fish

Once upon a time, From the time I was nearly nothing, I got looks at my grandpa.

Taking off into the forest promptly toward the beginning of the day prior to the sun had risen, at the point when a large portion of the world's occupants was not, in any case, starting to mix. He Would conveys a little pack, which I knew held a pencil and a scratchpad.

Sometimes I would see him coming back from the forest, pack close by, with a

Look of miracle all over. He would consistently get back in time for lunch,

What's more, my grandmother would have something yummy prepared for him.

At some point, when I was fourteen, Grandpa gave me a little bundle and said

"Grandson, take this scratch pad and pencil. Some early morning, before the daytime animals wake up yet after the nighttime animals have hit the sack, discover a spot somewhere down in the forest where you can sit and watch the forest as it Wakes from sleep. Utilize this pencil and scratchpad to record what you see furthermore, hear."

I guaranteed Grandpa I would do as he proposed. I had never observed what he had composed without anyone else scratchpad, yet I generally thought it must be the interesting stories he would tell Grandma and me. Since I had been given a scratch pad and pencil, I concluded I would compose astounding things simply like him!

It was a pre-winter before I got the chance to visit the forest. It was a crisp morning, yet not chilly, so I could stroll along with the ways without making a sound. I had no clue where I ought to go, so I just pushed further also, more profound into the forest. At last, I understood the animals would likely start waking soon. I saw a major pine tree and took a seat at the base, my back against the storage compartment, watching out at a little glade.

I could faintly hear running water and speculated that a stream was close by. I took my scratchpad and pencil from my pack and looked them over carefully in the diminishing light. With astonishing velocity, the light became more splendid and more brilliant.

I before long saw the sun's beams stimulating the highest points of the trees around the glade.

Someplace far above me, an early-rising squirrel unstuck a pinecone, and I tuned in to it ricochet from branch to branch as it tumbled from the tree I was sitting under, at long last landing delicately close to me. Indeed, even as I made a note of this on my scratchpad, I understood I would not have the option to compose stories as superb as my grandpa's. Yet, I kept on pausing and watch.

Winged creatures are consistently the first to alert, and soon I could hear them singing their morning tunes as they respected the sun and the new day. Feathered creatures shuddered to a great extent through the trees. The forest was, at last, waking up!

Right then and there, I felt exceptionally warm and understood a beam of the sun was painting me with its brilliant light.

It felt pleasant. It made me sleepy, yet I was resolved to remain alarmed to Watch the forest wrap awakening from the difficult night.

All of a sudden, I saw a development close to the edge of the glade. Something was weaving through the trees. Before long, I saw it was a deer'" a buck'" with a huge set of prongs on his head.

He was heavenly with his crown, resembling the ruler of the forest as he intrepidly ventured out onto the knoll.

He was in a mind-blowing prime: solid and sure, certain about his each

Step, realizing each stable that contacted him. I watched him take silently.

Steps, delaying once in a while as his ready ears moved and turned, getting all the forest sounds.

"This is awesome!" I contemplated it internally. Be that as it may, I didn't set out a move to compose any of this down. I realized the deer would leave on the off chance that he realized I was observing

him, so I sat still, scarcely in any event, relaxing.
Mindfully he crossed to the opposite side of the glade close to where the stream
was streaming. He glanced around, and his ears were exceptionally bustling jerking this
way and that. At the point when he was sure there was no risk, he plunged his head down to take his morning drink.
At that exact instant, when he had plunged his head down, the most intense sound I had ever heard emitted from the stream. The buck jumped into the air, ensnaring his fine prongs in the tree limbs overhead. He hung up there for a second or two, flailing wildly before he loosened up, fell to the ground, and afterward immediately limited away into the forest, never to be seen once more.

I hopped to my feet at the noisy sound, dropping my pack, pencil, and scratchpad. My heart was dashing, its sound beating in my ears. Be that as it may, the entire forest had gone quiet. I remained there quite a while, letting my heart slow down, thinking about what I ought to do straight away.

It occurred to me: my grandpa would head toward the stream where the deer had been to research the clamor. I couldn't allow my grandpa to down, trembling with dread and fervor, I got my things and went unobtrusively, `indeed, even stealthily, over the knoll to where the deer had halted to drink.

I arrived at the stream and glanced carefully around me. Despite the fact that I proved unable to jerk my ears from side to side, despite everything, I listened eagerly for anything abnormal. A couple of feathered creatures had started to sing once more. An intermittent breeze stirred through the, for the most part, stripped trees. The stream murmured delicately before me.

Following a couple of moments of simply remaining there, I concluded I would take a beverage from the rivulet before recording what I had seen and heard that morning.

I carefully ventured to the edge of the water. A school of fish had a break in the spring, and the idea entered my thoughts to bring my fishing Shaft next time. As I bowed down toward the water, one fish quickly rose toward me. Just before my lips arrived at the water, the fish sprung up and clearly, noisily, stronger than anything I had ever heard, stated,

"Hello!"

The sound and stun, all things considered, made me slip and fall. My legs got wet when I entered the stream, and my hands and garments got all sloppy as I immediately crept up the bank. My ears were ringing as I ran right over the knol to the pine tree, where I tossed myself down at its delicate base once more. I lay there for quite a while, attempting to make sense of what I had recently seen.

At last, I sat up once more, pulled my pencil and scratch pad from my pack, and carefully composed what I had seen and heard that day. My arms and legs started to dry in the warm sun. As I was writing in my scratchpad, I was eager to acknowledge I was composing a story nearly as unfathomable as one of my grandpa's! I rushed to complete, pressed my things, and unobtrusively left the forest.

It was a long stroll back to Grandpa's place, which made me hungry. At the point when I left the forested areas, Grandpa was perched on the yard watching me. We have taken a gander at one another purposely. I could see he realized that I currently knew something curious and exceptional about the forest. And afterward, he stated,

"Grandson, your grandmother has made a fine lunch of potato soup with natively constructed buns. Why not go along with us?"

Obviously, I did. No one left behind Grandma's buns. While we ate, I told them a stunning story that couldn't in any way, shape, or form be valid. At the point when lunch was over,

Grandpa took a gander at me genuine hard, at that point winked. I winked back at Grandpa and stated, "A debt of gratitude is in order for the notebook and pencil."

His eyes shone, and he gestured his head. At that point, I pardoned myself to go home and sleep. It had been a difficult day as of now!

Good night

8. The fish who could peruse

Sheila was the most stunning fish in the sea, and therefore, numerous other fish and seas animals had an aversion for her.

"She's so occupied," the octopus would state as they drifted about drinking tea." Why wouldn't she be able to be still and eat seaweed?"

For the most part, sea animals got a kick out of the chance to move with the waves, and in light of the fact that Sheila had a robot tail and blades, she wasn't keen on rolling. She liked to swim as fast as possible. She realized she was a touch of a pariah to the more seasoned fishes and such; however, she couldn't support herself.

Furthermore, she had one companion who wanted to invest energy with her regardless of how fast or far or careless she swam.

Starry, the starfish, was something contrary to Sheila, the robot fish. When Sheila hustled, Starry lay still. When Sheila dove, Starry lay still. When Sheila spiraled through logs at the base of the sea, Starry lay still. However consistently, Sheila advanced toward Starry's sandy floor, and consistently, Starry anticipated it.

"The octopus pack was especially frantic at me today Starry," the robot fish disclosed to her companion, and she orbited her star molded companion. "I do feel somewhat awful about spilling a portion of their tea. However, it's an in the sea, and there's in every case parts to drink."

"I wouldn't stress over them, Sheila, and they're generally so cranky."

Sheila could generally depend on Starry to urge her to do what she cherished best, which obviously was to do anything she desired. Furthermore, as an approach to state thank you for that, she needed to accomplish something pleasant for Starry.

"Starry, in the event that you could have one astonishment, what might you need it to be?"

"I'd need somebody to peruse me the Harry Potter books. I've heard such a great amount about the Harry Potter books. However, I don't know any individual who can peruse. Or, on the other hand, any individual who has them and who in the event that they had them would have the option to peruse to me."

"All robots can peruse Starry, and I could do that for you."

"Truly, Sheila. You would peruse for me?"

"Unquestionably, and I know a submerged ship that has the Harry Potter books on them."

Sheila swam fiercely all through a wide range of schools of fish that would, in general, assemble for water cooler talk each evening.

"Heads up!" hollered some fish. "You're insane!" shouted a swell fish. "You're going to catch your tail in a net!" a dolphin squeaked. Be that as it may, Sheila held swimming to the wrecked books. At that point, she swam some increasingly, upsetting more crabs and fish and talking seaweed as she went.

The sea animal network had enough, and as Sheila dashed by, they gradually pursued.

"Okay, Starry, I have the book." And Sheila started perusing. It was the most delightful thing the little starfish had ever heard. For five minutes, her robot fish companion hovered still in the water, perusing page after page.

At last, the other sea animals made up for the lost time to Sheila and were going to voice their serious disappointment on how troublesome her fast swimming was to their apathetic days. In any case, as they arranged to do as such, they excessively got spellbound by the story.

You may realize that, alongside being famously against fast and uncontrollable swimmers, sea animals are likewise unfit to peruse. As they watched Sheila reveal to her tale, they, at last, acknowledged how extraordinary this robot fish was. For four hours, they all hovered unobtrusively, just some of them taking breaks to arrive at the surface so they could breathe. Sheila didn't break once and didn't stop to perceive what number of individuals were in her crowd. She read to Starry just as she was the just one around.

"What's more, that is the finish of the first Harry Potter book," she said at long last, shutting the books enlarged pages. It was at exactly that point that Sheila saw ho numerous individuals had been tuning in. "Goodness, hello there everyone," she stated, and afterward went right back to swimming uncontrollably, shooting all through schools of fish.

Be that as it may, no one halted her, and no one hollered. Rather, gradually, the other fish started to swim heedlessly, until you could see just a haze of air pockets up and down the seafloor.
"Yahoo for Sheila, the perusing robot fish!" shouted the octopus. What's more, starting there on, no one was ever made a decision for being too energized again.

9. The City Under The Sea

Sometime in the distant past, in a nation of mountains which flanked upon the sea, abided a rich vendor who had three children. The oldest and the second-conceived were his delights, for they were traders as well and stayed next to him; however, the youngest regularly caused him much anxiety. Not so, this youngest child was a wild or a terrible fellow, yet the love of the sea and want for experience ran like fire in his veins, and he couldn't force himself to sit close to his dad and his siblings in the checking house.

Tired finally of the steady censures of his family, he dismissed one night from his dad's home and joined a ship as a typical mariner. Clad in mariner blue, wearing a little top, a pullover open at the throat, and pants cut wide at the bottoms, the runaway chap cruised over the sea to remote terrains and isles. What's more, as the years passed, individually, and brought no greetings of him, his dad and his siblings surrendered him for lost.

Presently the King of the nation wherein the rich dealer and his child stayed adored uncommon pearls and valuable stones more than everything else on the planet. Covered up furtively away in the profound establishments of his manor lay his fortune room: it was roundabout fit as a fiddle and worked of dark marble, and at equivalent separation one from the other, along the bending divider, stood a hundred statues of equipped men, holding consistently consuming lights. A hundred coffers of greenstone lay on the floor, one at the base of every statue, every coffer heaped high with diamonds.

After quite a while after night, when all was still, the King would slide to the mystery chamber, and tossing open the covers of the gem chests, would look long and quietly into the shining mass inside.

One night the King drove his neighbor, the Emperor of the Seven Isles, to the gem room, and gave him his fortunes.

"Are there more attractive gems to be found in the entire world?" said the King gladly.

"They are as a general rule decent," addressed the Emperor, signaling his dim head. "In any case, how happens it that the Emerald of the Sea isn't among them? The Emerald, is a creature of the Sea and it is the most brilliant jewel in the whole world. A long time back, an angler of the Land of the Dawn found it in a strangely cut box that a whirlwind had washed into his nets. I saw it when I was all things considered a youthful ruler.

Where can we find the emerald, asked the King, who was overwhelmed with the yearning to add the jewel to his benefits? "Tell me that I may promptly send a battle looking for it."

"I have not thought about it for around, an exhausting year," addressed the Emperor, "notwithstanding, it is still in the Dawn land.

So remarkable was the King's tension to transform into the owner of the Emerald of the Sea, that he could scarcely keep things under control for the initial segment of the day. For the duration of the night, he rested, not a wink for thinking about it, and scarcely had the red shield of the morning sun rose above the petite mists lying at the edge of the ocean and sky when he sent for the rich seller to go to the imperial living arrangement at once.

Contemplating much at the solicitation, the seller made whirlwind to the imperial living arrangement and was there taken rapidly before the King. Right when the King saw him, he said:–

"You are the best and most indulgent seller in my spaces. Know, by then, that I have an endeavor meriting you. Then, in the Land of the Dawn, there is a diamond called the Emerald of the Sea; it is your endeavor to find it and get it for me. To have it, I would give all the gold in my space. Notice that you return with it.

The merchant bowed low and addressed that he might want that very day sail for the Land of the Dawn in his quickest ship. By then, getting back, he gave orders that the best vessel in the total of his naval forces be immediately masterminded the experience; subsequently immediately was this done, the seller traveled for the Land of the Dawn in the first part of the day tide.

Numerous days and numerous classes, he cruised, over sparkling seas, till he arrived at the harbor of the Land of the Dawn. Boats were entering, and ships were leaving the dazzling mountain-surrounded narrows. How the expansive sails pulled at their ropes as a relentless breeze filled their bending white profundities! How silver-clear shone the wrinkles of froth streaming back from the forward rushing bows!

Advancing out toward the incredible, still, a reflection of the mid-year sea, was a peculiar dark vessel, with sails as red as fire.

The vendor tied down his ship in a peaceful narrows and rushed aground to discover the Lord Treasurer of the Kingdom. He discovered this aristocrat calm on a gallery of his stronghold, which overlooked the sea. After hearing the dealer's story, the aristocrat started with shock, and said:–

"You are simply past the point of no return! At the direction of my regal ace, the Prince of the Land of the Dawn, I sold the Emerald of the Sea just an hour prior to the ace of an abnormal vessel. It couldn't be any more obvious, and there she is present." And the Lord Treasurer called attention to over the sea to the dark ship with the red sails, which was simply then vanishing over the skyline.

Grateful that the other ship was still in locate, the vendor rushed back to his very own vessel and gave pursue. rFortunately for him, there was a full moon that night, by which the shadowy mass and the influencing poles of the puzzling boat could be seen.

All the following day, they cruised, yet never an inch closer to the next vessel did they come. However, the shipper stacked his ship with all the canvas she could bear. One more night and one more day discovered them no closer. At last, late toward the evening of the third day, an incredible tempest came cruising over the edge of the sea; an impact of wind struck the shipper's ship, at that point a downpour of the downpour, and the night went ahead similarly as the tempest was at its tallness.

At the point when the sunshine came back again, the other ship had totally vanished; and however, the stressed trader cruised here and cruised there, never an indication of the outsider might he be able to discover. Finally, with overwhelming sadness, he surrendered the mission and came back to his King with the malicious news.

The King, I scarcely need to say, was next to himself with wrath and dissatisfaction. Frowning so horribly that his eyebrows nearly met, he cried to the shipper:–

"Fraud, through you, I have lost the best gem on the planet! eOn the off chance that you don't discover it inside a year, your life and your assets will be relinquished to me."

On hearing these horrendous words, the shipper turned pale, for he had no more thought where the Emerald of the Sea can be found than had another conceived child. His two children, in any case, when they had heard his story, bade him not to surrender and proclaimed that they would that very night go forward and look for the emerald through the world.

Presently, in light of the fact that the poor dealer couldn't stand to be disregarded very, it was, at last, concurred that solitary the oldest child ought to go in search of the gem, while the second-conceived ought to stay at home. This, obviously, was much against the desire of the subsequent child; by the by, so it was organized.

Thus the oldest child cruised away. tThe days stretched into weeks, the weeks into months, the months into a year, yet the oldest child didn't return. A gatekeeper of troopers drove the troubled trader before the King.

"All things considered, have you discovered the Emerald of the Sea?" said the King.

"No," answered the dealer, pitifully. Furthermore, presently all would positively have been over with the poor vendor, had not his subsequent child asked and begged the King for a time of relief wherein he, as well, may search for the emerald through the world. In spite of the fact that from the start reluctant, the King finally respected the request, however, he demanded one portion of the shipper's assets as a relinquish.

Thus the subsequent child cruised away. Days stretched into weeks, weeks protracted into months, the months into a year, yet the subsequent child didn't return. Pitiless tempests destroyed such a large number of the vendor's ships that he lost the other portion of his assets, and had to take shelter in a hopeless bungalow by the swamps past the town.

On the most recent night of the year allowed to him by the King, the troubled man sat in his poor abode by a disintegrating driftwood fire, tuning in to the surf breaking on the seashore that edged the bog. Far away, he heard the chimes of the illustrious city sound the 12 PM hour. Neither the oldest child nor the second-conceived had returned. The second year of rest was at an end; nothing presently could remain the displeasure of the King.

Abruptly there came a vivacious rodent tat-tat on the entryway.

"I am lost," mumbled the poor trader to himself. "The King's troopers are as of now at the entryway." And progressing insecurely over the room, he tossed the entryway open wide.
A whirlwind from the sea blew in, which twisted back the fire of the decrease in his grasp, and afterward, over the limit ventured the youngest child. He was as yet a mariner and clad in mariner blue, and there was a cutlass in his belt. So shaken with delight was the trader that for quite a while, he couldn't express a word, yet simply clung to the solid shoulders of the young seaman.

Concerning the mariner child, he figured out how to tell his dad that he had come back from far off grounds just that very night, and had recently known about the fiascos h overtaken his family.

As they were talking, walking steps were heard outside; and afterward, without holding back to thump, a sergeant of the King's watchman constrained open the entryway and, trailed by a bunch of officers, went into the pitiable room and took the trader and his child detainees. They went through the night on the straw in the regal cells, and in the first part of the day were driven before the King.

On observing the shipper, the perturbed King frowned more irately than any time in recent memory,– for the loss of the Emerald of the Sea had never quite disturbed him,– and said:–

"All things considered, have you discovered the Emerald of the Sea?"

"No," said the poor shipper.

"Gather the killer!" cried the King.

What's more, presently, the poor man would absolutely have bid goodbye to earth, had not the youngest child, similar to his siblings, intervened with the King.

From the start, the King would hear not an expression of it, and called to his gatekeeper to take the detainees right away; yet it being murmured that the mariner, despite the fact that very little in excess of a chap, had once battled intrepidly and been painfully injured in the illustrious help, he finally offered ear to the youngest child's supplication and said:–

"Truly, you will have one more year. However, I realize that this year will be the last. In the event that you don't come back with the Emerald of the Sea inside a twelvemonth, nothing will spare you. I have spoken."

Also, subsequently, the mariner child went in search of the Emerald. What befell him upon his search, in what circumstance he discovered his siblings, and how he visited the City under the Sea, you will without further ado hear.

Presently the youngest child had his very own little pontoon. It was little to such an extent that, when the breeze never again filled its sails, it could be paddled along, and in this vessel, the mariner chap started his journey. From the harbor to harbor, from country to country, he cruised, yet never a spirit he discovered who could reveal to him nothing of the weird dark ship with the blazing sails or the lost Emerald of the Sea. Indeed, even the individuals of the Land of the Dawn could reveal to him just that the diamond had been offered to an obscure sovereign.

By and by the winter of the year overtook him, and in one of the abrupt tempests that proclaimed the happening to the cool, his little vessel went shorewards on a rough coast and was before the long beat to pieces by the breakers. Tossed into the sea during the disaster area, the mariner was himself so hurled and stomped on by the waves that he arrived at the shore unmistakably more dead than alive. Surely, had it not been for a poor fisherman and his significant other, there would have been no more story to tell. These great individuals, I am happy to state, protected the mariner from the anger of the waters, and breastfed him back to wellbeing and quality once more.

At the point when his quality was very reestablished, the mariner recounted to this great couple the story of how he had gone forward to look for through the wide world the Emerald of the Sea.

"In any case, my poor fellow," said the benevolent fisherman, "the Emerald of the Sea has always evaporated from mortal eyes."

"What! You are aware of the emerald?" cried the mariner.

"Tsk-tsk, yes," answered the fisherman. "Two years prior to the Prince of the Unknown Isles sent the best vessel in his armada to the Land of the Dawn to purchase the gem. An excellent ship was she, with a body as pitch dark and sails as red as fire. My sibling and I cruised in her group. The gem was taken on board. Our fearless ship set sail for the Unknown Isles. Scarcely were we three days out of seeing the area, when a tempest overtook us and sank the vessel. I risked to be hurled in the water close to an extraordinary part of the pole aand clung to this until a passing vessel discovered me. Of all on board, only I endure. Forty understands profound falsehoods the Emerald of the Sea, never more to be seen yet by the moronic animals of the waters."

At these greetings the daring mariner's heart became like ice; by the by, he cried:–

"Tsk-tsk, great companion, I realize that what you state is valid, yet will I not surrender; for, come what will, I should spare my dad!"

Hearing this, the fisherman's significant other, a tranquil, decent body who had wanted to sit quiet, murmured that it would be well first to counsel the Witch of the Sands.

"The Witch of the Sands? Who is she, and where would I be able to discover her?" cried the mariner.

"The Witch of the Sands stays a hundred groups from here," answered the fisherman's significant other. "Every one of the riddles of the waters is in her keeping, and she has a response for them all. You should go to her and request her assistance, you."

So the mariner expressed gratitude toward the great fisherman and his better half and set out to walk a hundred associations to the place of the Witch of the Sands. His way lay along with a destroy and forlorn shore, on whose rough seashores the wooden bones of old wrecks lay spoiling, half-covered in stones and weed. Similarly, as the third day's sun was soaking in the sparkling waters, the mariner landed at the Witch's residence.

The Witch made her home in a left old ship, which a tempest of some time in the past had thrown far up the sands. With respect to the Witch herself, she was a lady so old that the mariner idea she without a doubt more likely than not been living when the moon and the stars were made. An edge of sea-shells circumnavigated the crown of her high cap, and round her wrists were wrist trinkets of silvery periwinkles.

Similarly, as the mariner moved toward the Witch's entryway, a young hide seal, who had been lolling in a little pool left along the seashore by the tide, rushed out of his puddle, and running quickly toward him on his flappers, cuddled his hand with his smooth, wet head, much the same as a young canine.

"Down, Neptune, down!" cried the witch abrasively.

"Goodbye, madam," said the mariner in his politest way.

"You are the third individual who has come here to ask me the inquiry you will solicit," shouted the Witch of the Sands, whose enchantment powers had uncovered to her the explanation of the mariner's coming. "I know you! You are the youngest child. Your two siblings have been here to ask me the route under the sea, and I let them know; however favor me, they have n't returned yet. Much the same as young men to overlook an elderly person's admonition. I have got a decent personality not to reveal to you the route to the under-waters; without a doubt, I would n't participate in the event that you were n't a mariner and a child of the sea. Indeed, I can show you the way to under the sea; yet you should not get some information about the emerald since I don't have a clue swhere it is myself. In the Land of the Dawn, and that is the last I thought about it! Exactly when you do get to the under-waters, recollect that. You'll have to hustle back like a breeze for the year, which the King gave your father is about gone. Do whatever it takes not to ask me requests! I understand you will ask one since I'm not a man, and I perceive what you will solicit, considering the way that I'm á witch."

Besides, the unusual, elderly person laughed and, putting her hands on her midsection, impacted so ruthlessly from side to side that the shells on her top shook and clicked. By then, after a postponement to aggregate breath, she continued: "Before you can go down into the waters, I should give you a spellbound ring. There are three of them in the whole world, and your kin have the other two. Goodness, me, be that as it may, I don't have the foggiest thought why I let them take my charm rings. Since I actually, I don't know as I will let you take my ring. Regardless, it has been at the front line of my musings for a long time to tell their King under the Sea that he's been encouraging the tide to stop overall excessively near my ship.
There was a relief, and the sailor, who had checked out the entirety of Witch's words, gravely promised to pass on her message to the King under the Sea. He was going to represent a request or two, when the Witch of the Sands, drawing another long, long breath, yelled out again:–

"Do whatever it takes not to present requests! I've told you once, and I've revealed to you twice, and I'll tell you indistinguishable number of times from there are drops of water in the ocean! The route to the City under the Sea begins a hundred classes toward the north; in the high feigns there, when the tide is low, you'll find the mouth of an amazing natural hollow; walk around this sinkhole, and further and additionally further and further down, till you feel water climbing around your feet. By then, put on my ring and walk emphatically ahead. In a brief timeframe, you will see the city shimmering in the waters. Once there, search out the King and let him know about your voyage.

10.The Witch took from a little

Calfskin satchel a straightforward brilliant ring and gave it to the youngest child, who put the ring in his pocket, expressed gratitude toward the Witch, and set off for the cave, which prompted the City under the Sea. You might be certain it didn't take him exceptionally long to discover it.
In the wake of feeling careful in his pocket to check whether the ring was as yet sheltered, the mariner dove on into the winding cavern.

In a brief timeframe, the thunder of the breakers on the seashore, which had been uproarious at the mouth of the sinkhole, started to blur and develop swoon, and the passage developed dim and cold. Feeling for the mass of the entry with one hand, the youngest child progressed into the obscurity. Animals of the sea, with round sparkling eyes, stared at him from shallow pools, and once in a while, his hand, running along the wall, would touch and shake from its place a starfish or great snail.
Further and further down and down went the mariner. By and by, he heard the lapping of wavelets in the dimness, and a couple of moments after, he felt himself progressing into extending water. Halting for a moment, he put on the brilliant ring. At that point, strolling on once more, he felt the

water ascend from his lower legs to his abdomen, and from his midsection to his throat. One stage more, and the water shut over his head.

Once under the waves, the mariner wavered, dubious with respect to what direction to turn. Gradually, in any case, his eyes became used to the bit of the water, and he saw, lying on the last a couple of feet in front of him, a little ball sparkling with a pale glowing light. Going as far as to contact this peculiar article, the mariner discovered it to be a little round sea-plant which had tied down itself to stone, and directly he discovered that this light was nevertheless one of the thousands which together framed a long straight line over the level floor of the sea. Properly envisioning these lights to be indications of a sea-world street, the mariner progressed along with them. A moderate stroll of ten long classes carried him to the entryway of the City under the Sea.

There was next to no light there, put something aside for that which got through the waters from the planet, and this was nevertheless a blackout, light green sparkle.
The mariner strolled unchallenged through the door and wound up in the incredible road of the city. Along the wide road developed goliath sea-plants with darker leaves, set out in lines like trees; and through the foliage which moved intensely in the flows, little fish shot like flying creatures. Numerous individuals strolled gradually back and forth abnormal individuals of the sea, and all dressed the same in tight-fitting pieces of clothing of sparkling, fish-like scales.

The mariner investigated their countenances and saw that a brilliant wide ring circled the understudies of their eyes. All of a sudden, two men of the sea, recognized from the others by swords of red stone, traveled through the water and holding onto the mariner in their webbed hands, rushed him before the King of the Under-Waters.

On a coral honored position, in an incredible corridor roofed with a high roundabout vault, sat the King. The streaming waters inside were splendid, and an eccentric, light green light punctured through the lobby from a sort of wellspring of light in the focal point of the floor under the arch. Moving toward this sparkling wellspring, the mariner discovered it to be a mass of shining sea-animals, living blooms of the profound, which, even as he looked, blended their puzzling petals.

"Welcome, Wearer and the bearer of the Enchanted Ring," said the King, staring hard at the mariner with his enormous brilliant eyes. "You come at a blessed time. This very night we commend the wedding of the second of my three girls with the human wearer of the subsequent ring. Stand you upon the means of the royal position, for they are coming immediately. Allow the trumpets to sound!"

In this direction, two young people of the sea lifted gigantic conch-shells to their mouths and sounded them.

Extraordinary entryways in a split second opened wide, and a dazzling parade entered. To begin with, seemed twelve pages; at that point, in strolled the Sea King's subsequent little girl, connected at the hip with a joyful young man, in whom the mariner perceived his second-most established sibling.

Directly the conch-shells sounded once more.

11.The Princess and the Prince cried out a voice.

The King hung-over from his royal position and murmured in the mariner's ear:–

"My oldest girl and her better half. They were hitched only a year back. The Prince is a young people of the world above, and wears the first of the charming rings."

Presently entered the oldest Princess of the Sea, strolling by the side of her better half. Also, in the spouse, the young mariner observed the senior of his two siblings. Also, however, the young mariner loosened up his arms to them, neither of his siblings recollected that him, for a while blackout and hungry, they had overlooked the admonition of the Witch and had eaten OUT OFthe bread of the under-world. In this way had the memory of the world over, the lost emerald, and their dad's predicament blurred away.

The conches sounded a third time.

"Go to the wedding dinner," cried the King. "You will sit next to my youngest little girl."

Furthermore, presently the mariner chap, helter-skelter, was rushed into the meal corridor and seated at the illustrious table alongside the King's youngest little girl. Furthermore, she was an incredible, generally excellent of all the three. Seeing that the youngest child contacted no nourishment, she said to him:–

"For what reason do you won't taste of the wedding feast?"

"Princess," answered the mariner, "I have gone to the Under-Waters to look for the Emerald of the Sea; for in the event that I come back to my own nation without it, my dad's life will be relinquished. Okay, have me overlook?"

"Be that as it may, you will never discover the Emerald of the Sea!" cried the Princess.

"Never discover the Emerald of the Sea! What do you mean?" said the mariner restlessly.

"The Emerald of the Sea has vanished," proceeded with the little Princess, fixing the mariner with her brilliant eyes. "Years back, it was taken from my dad's treasury by a fiendish Prince of the Under-Waters. My dad sought after him and overthrew him, yet in the battle, the emerald was lost, and ascending to the surface, floated to the shores of the Land of the Dawn. There it stayed till the Prince of the Unknown Isles bought it and removed it in his dark ship. This ship, overcome by a tempest, sank, yet where it lies we know not. Whosoever discovers it will be ace of the land under the sea, for the emerald is ace of every one of us. My dad won't lift a finger to assist you with discovering it; to be sure, on the off chance that he realizes that you are in search of it, he will drive you to eat out of the bread of the under-waters. State nothing, along these lines, of your mission."

At these words, the bold mariner's heart sank extremely low. Mindful of the Witch's notice, he challenged contact no piece of nourishment, yet he realized that yearning would before long acquire shortcoming its train. Possibly he should discover the emerald without a moment's delay, or he should forsake all expectation of discovering it. He couldn't live long in the event that he contacted no nourishment, and if, however, one piece contacted his lips, he would overlook the upper world.

Far away, the poor trader, whom the King had now thrown in jail, viewed the days pass individually, and the most recent year approaches its end. Each morning he would request greetings of his mariner child and ask futile.

Presently, when the wedding feast was over, and the ball which pursued was at its stature, the oldest of the princesses called her sister, the lady of the hour, aside and said to her:–

"We should free ourselves on the double of this newcomer. I observed him loosen up his arms to them as they passed. Who can tell yet that he may lead them away from us? Let us advise our workers to lie in sit tight for him and convey us from such a threat."

So said the oldest sister, of the brilliant eyes. Oh, I dread that the individuals of the under-waters are sometimes very as stunning as those of the world above.

Later that night, similarly as poor people mariner was remaining by one of the extraordinary entryways, twelve or so heavy rebels in the administration of the oldest sister fell upon him, bound him with lines, and hauled him through the water to the illustrious stables.

Presently the individuals of the under-waters, having no ponies– for sea steeds are nevertheless modest animals– had subdued extraordinary dolphins to convey them about. Hundreds of the monsters, each with a bronze ring in his nose, were run at the edges of the stables, and on the fiercest and angriest of all, the Princess' hirelings tied the mariner. How the extraordinary fish, fastened to a bar by a chain and his nose-ring, pulled, rolled, swerved aside, and whipped his tail! However, every one of his twisting's was of no profit, for the poor mariner fellow was before long fastened to his back with a rope of seaweed. At that point, the animal was discharged from his chain, given a blow as an afterthought with a whip of shark-skin, and transformed into the wilds of the under-waters.
For thirty minutes, the fish, startled at his weight, fled at lightning speed over the tops of the city into the forlorn plain. At that point, stopping his frantic flight, he attempted again to shake himself liberated from the mariner. He turned, he jumped, he plunged, yet all futile, for the mariner was safely fastened to his back. Alarmed over again, with a quick movement of his incredible balances, he shot fiercely to the other side and hurried endlessly into the dim. Throughout the entire that night, he fled. Close to the morning of the following day, in any case, the mariner figured out how to function one arm free, and draw the cutlass from his midsection. The incredible animal, conveyed of the weight which had lain upon it, rose on the tip of its tail and shot frantically toward the surface, and the mariner tumbled through the waters to the base.
Powerless and hungry, the poor young seaman looked about in the half-unhappiness and wound up on the lower slants of a depressed mountain ascending from the seafloor. Toward no path would he be able to locate an indication of the City under the Sea. Trusting, nonetheless, to see better

from the peak, he chose to climb it. Weird plants and shells lay in the cleft of the weedy rocks, schools of brilliant fish fled past him like living bolts, and tremendous crabs left away as he showed up. All of a sudden, lying on her side in a little gorge of the mountain, he saw a ship–the dark ship of the Emerald of the Sea! Exhausted and frail however he was, it took the mariner yet a minute to climb on board, and rush past the wrecked poles into the skipper's lodge. A consistent, green brilliance shone in one corner of the weedy room and hurrying toward it, the mariner found, finally, the Emerald of the Sea. The crate which had walled it in had spoiled away and self-destructed.

"Triumph!" cried the mariner, "a triumph! The emerald is mine finally, and I will spare my dad."

He took the extraordinary gem from the messed up confine and rested it the cup of his two hands how it gleamed on the pale tissue! At that point, pushing it into a pocket and clutching it with one hand, he rushed out again to the mountainside.

On the planet above, it was high early afternoon, and the level beams of the sun beat profound into the green waters. So splendid had the incline become, that the mariner chap felt sure that he couldn't be a long way from the outside of the waves. Moreover, if the peak transcended the waters, it would frame an island in the upper world. Thus, without a doubt, it was. Jumping on toward the highest point of the mountain, the mariner previously scaled a precarious precipice, and at the highest point of this, he found a delicate incline of sand. The sun's beams presently lit up the water so splendidly that the air appeared to be just a little separation away. By and by, a seashore crab fled from underneath the mariner's feet. The water became especially hotter. The shore was close by! A couple of steps more, and the youngest child developed on the seashore of an excellent isle.

Half-blinded by the sun, he strolled toward the dry land. There he discovered some delightful organic products developing and an undulating stream of precious stone water. He ate and drank, and his quality returned.

Himself once more, the mariner took the Emerald of the Sea in his grasp, and cried,–

"By the intensity of the Emerald of the Sea, I bring here the two senior princesses of the under-waters, and my two siblings, their spouses!"

There was a sound of far roar under the reasonable blue sky, and after a minute, four heads emerged from the waters and shaking the salt splash from their eyes, the princesses and the siblings strolled through the shallows to where the mariner was standing. Presently, the princesses were particularly alarmed when they observed the mariner holding the almighty emerald, and falling on their knees before him, beseeched him to excuse their offenses, and not to remove their friends and family. Tears tumbled from their brilliant eyes and blended with the drops of the salty sea as yet coursing down their dark scales. Concerning the siblings, they would have heaved themselves upon the mariner, had not the enchantment power of the emerald forestalled their methodology.

"Be kind and pardon," said the younger of the sisters. "All things considered, had we not made you be energetic away, you would never have discovered the emerald."

"Indeed, that is valid," said the mariner. "My siblings will choose for themselves. Break, at that point, the spell which ties them to the under-waters, reestablishes to them their memory of the past, and in the event that, at that point, they decide to remain, I will make an effort not to lead them away. Invert the spell!"

"That is effectively done," said the senior sister. "Let them, however, contact the nourishment or drink of the upper world, and their memory will return."

What's more, in less time than it takes to tell it, the sisters offered the charmed siblings water from the current. At the point when they had smashed of it, both the siblings got horribly washed out, their eyes were wide opened, and they stared as peculiarly as men abruptly waked from sleep. At that point, seeing their younger sibling, they raced to him and tossed their arms about him, and posed a thousand inquiries about their dad and the journey of the emerald.

The brilliant peered toward ladies watched them with miserable appearances, lastly, broke into calm tears. Envision their bliss, when their spouses came back to them and bade them be of optimism.

Therefore was genuine affection seen as mightier than the mightiest spell.

Presently, when the princesses of the sea had dried their tears, the mariner and his siblings consulted to how the Emerald of the Sea may be brought to the King in time to spare their dad's life. You may make a decision of the mariner's shock when he discovered that in view of an awful blunder in the schedules and timekeepers of Sixes and Sevens (a city he had visited as he continued looking for the emerald), the life of his dad had been relinquished to the King three days prior!

In any case, presently, we should come back to the poor shipper himself.

The poor man had lain in a little cell in the illustrious prisons, standing by tensely, gracious, so restlessly, to hear the brisk advance of the mariner child on the winding stairs simply outside his jail entryway. However, the year reached a conclusion, as you probably are aware, without his arrival. For the third and last time, the stronghold monitors drove the poor man before the King. Presently the King had never excused the dealer for the loss of the gem; his shame, in fact, had expanded with the years, and he was happy that he could finally render his retribution.

"Have you discovered the Emerald of the Sea?" said the King, cruelly. He stood erect on the means of his judgment-seat, arms collapsed, eyes fixed in a wild, dark scowl.

"No," said the dealer, discreetly.

"At that point, you will look for it yourself," cried the King. Furthermore, he gave orders that the shipper is tied hand and foot, and hurled into a little vessel without nourishment or drink, and afterward sent hapless to kick the bucket weakly in the desolate seas. Thus this terrible sentence was done.

Bound hand and foot, rare ready to move from side to side, the trader lay unmoving in his little art and stared up at the blue sky. By and by a forgiving sleep overcame him, and keeping in mind that he dozed, a breeze emerged, which cleared the little pontoon alongside it.

Then, on the delightful island, the mariner and his buddies, dazed at their discovery, started arrangements to come back to the under-waters. Similarly, as the dusk fell, all strolled together to the edge of the obscuring sea and progressed into the waves.

All of a sudden, the mariner, whose eyes were the quickest, saw a little vessel quickly floating shoreward. Presently trapped in an ebb and flow of the shallow seashore, it floated sideways; presently impelled by the rising tide, it drifted on, bow highlighted the shore. The mariner rushed toward it and held onto it. All of a sudden, he expressed a ringing cry! The old shipper lay on the floor of the pontoon. Despite everything, he lived, for they could see him tenderly relaxing. Lifting him up softly, the three children conveyed him to the shore, unloosed his bonds, and breathed life into him back.

Presently when the trader was himself once more, the mariner, through the intensity of the emerald, made the waves convey an incredible ship to the island, and on this ship, the three children, the two princesses, and the old shipper came back to the dealer's nation. All landed covertly, nonetheless, for they realized that the furious King would hold onto them on the off chance that he knew about their arrival. Thus it happened that, one night, not long after the homecoming, the word was brought to the mariner that the King had known about the dealer's break and was sending watchmen to capture the shipper and his buddies.

It was nearly 12 PM when the mariner chap got the admonition. Taking the emerald with him, he progressed to a window by the sea, and shouted out over the twilight waters, "Waters of the Sea, rise and overwhelm the castle of the King!"

Presently the King's castle stood separated independent from anyone else on a tongue of land running out of sight the tide, and soon the rising waters were streaming over the marble floors and pouring in through the windows. Individually, the lights in the thousand rooms, contacted by the waves, murmured, sputtered, and terminated. The hirelings of the royal residence, the whole gang, fled higgledy-piggledy and left the dim manor to its destiny. Gradually the propelling water crawled from the dividers to the galleries, from the overhangs to their exceptionally beat. At last, all the moon could see as it shone upon the flood was the climate vane of the most noteworthy turret of all. You ought to have seen the little waves wave and break about it! Lastly, even the climate vane vanished under the dark waves.
Secured his mystery treasure-room, opening the gem coffers in a steady progression, the King remained very uninformed of the debacle. For quite a while, no solid contacted him in his concealed retreat, in light of the fact that the entryway of the fortune room was extremely thick and solid. Abruptly he heard behind him the sound of falling water and moving in the direction of the entryway, observed surges of water spouting through the entries between the entryway and its casing. Frightfulness struck. He viewed the entryway burst from its locks and pivots; a thundering course of cold sea-water came pouring in the room, and after a minute, the entire manor disintegrated and self-destructed.

Presently, when the King had met his deserts, the individuals of the nation, who incredibly regarded the vendor, offered him the crown; however, he declined it and gave it on his two senior children. Hence it happened that the nation had two lords. Every sibling thusly ruled for a half year of consistently and spent the other six under the sea with the brilliant looked at individuals of the waters.

With respect to the mariner chap, he cruised the sea for a long time, lastly, wedded a niece of the Witch of the Sands. At that point, similar to all mariners, he went to the nation to live. His home is worked of dim stone, ivy moves over it, and apple plantations lie underneath its windows.

Also, they all lived cheerfully ever after.

12. PHILIP, THE SEA WOLF

Philip, the wicked sea wolf, is truly stressed. Sitting on the sand, advantages, he thinks and thinks. For what reason isn't the sky as blue as in the past? When was the last time that the seagull Vonda visited him? For what reason wouldn't he be able to swim free?

Previously, the sea was straightforward, and he could go fishing relaxed.

The experience of searching for nourishment was such a lot of fun! However, these days, who can get what they are searching for when everything is in such short stock?

The light is restricted; the sun's smell is constrained. Everything is restricted, with the exception of the dark stain that was brought into the world one morning and developed and developed in the sea. It is unappeasable, it eats the fish, fowls, and any individual who approaches endures a similar destiny.

The shore is unfilled, Philip looks despondent; A child's giggling isn't heard, and the music he loves isn't heard either. The planes don't quit flying overhead.

They assault the stain splashing liquid from the air. The old wolf, Nathan, has no answers. Not by any means, his mystery examinations can clarify what's happening.

Miss Candy, the uproarious mouthed seal, doesn't quit whining: "It isn't on the whole correct to make our skin so filthy! These stains can't be expelled by any means, what do you think?"

The sea isn't a junk receptacle, and baby wolves can't swim around alone and play in the waves, it isn't right!

The catfish, with its enormous mustache, let them know in his marine language that he was moving endlessly with his companions.

– "My home is totally pulverized; there is no chance to get out; there is no chance to get out!"

– "And, who can deal with this agonizing smell?" – hollered the stammering crab.

The stain will remain perpetually if the breeze doesn't blowhard. Numerous knick-knacks baby wolves started to move toward it. In the event that the deceptive dark stuff gets you, you will wind up brimming with oil. The individuals who know say that if people don't help you, the conceivable outcomes of proceeding to live are likewise restricted.

The little wolves risk losing their skin's assurance. Philip thinks and thinks each morning, searching for an answer, on the grounds that the human arrangement isn't adequate.

– "And I would prefer not to be a spoilsport yet they stay nearby with that plane showering whatever it is onto the stain and, well, they should be careful the stain doesn't eat the sky too!

But..who all of a sudden comes avoiding through the mists? ¿Is it her, or is it not? Truly! At long last! Seagull Vonda, the voyaging seagull, has brought a response in due order regarding sure.

– "I came. I came! I have news, and the South is perfect!"

Every one of the wolves applauded joyfully, aside from Nathan.

– "What's going on grandpa, aren't you glad?"

– "We, the most established, are moderate, on the off chance that we as a whole leave, who will look out for the shore?".

Philip's dark looked at stare submerged to the base of the sea, together with his expectations. Aa few weeks, and the island rocks are betrayed, the stain is the main visitor on the seashore.

A few kilometers away, the seagull Vonda has a troublesome activity. To manage those cumbersome, however, tenacious explorers. Her wingbeat is a moving expectation. The little wolf Philip is at the leader of the gathering as their commander, and he doesn't quit singing with the stammering crab a lo… lo… long melody.

Well, companions, I think I need to pack and go with them. Move, as people say. I like to state that I'm going to search for new expectations and new experiences.

13. The Rainbow Fish Story

Sometime in the distant past, far out in the dark blue sea, there carried on a fish. A normal fish, however, the most wonderful fish in the whole sea. His scales were each shade of blue and green and purple with shining silver scales among them. The other fish were astonished at his excellence. They called him 'Rainbow Fish.' "Please Rainbow Fish," they would call, "Come and play with us!" But the Rainbow Fish would simply skim past, glad and quiet, allowing his scales to scales.

At some point, a little blue fish trailed him. "Rainbow Fish," he called, "sit tight for me. If you don't mind, give me one of your sparkling scales. They are so magnificent, and you have such a significant number of." "You need me to give you one of my extraordinary scales? Who do you think you are? Escape from me," cried the Rainbow Fish. Stunned, the little blue fish swam away. He was so disturbed, he mentioned to every one of his companions what had occurred. Also, from that point on, nobody would have anything to do with the Rainbow Fish. They dismissed when he swam by.

What great were the amazing, gleaming scales with nobody to appreciate them? Presently, he was the loneliest fish in the whole sea. He chose to spill out his difficulties to the starfish. The Rainbow Fish asked, "I truly am wonderful. For what reason doesn't anyone like me?" "I can't answer that for you! I you go past the coral reef to a profound cavern, you'll locate the astute octopus. Perhaps she can support you!" answered the starfish.

The rainbow fish found the cavern. It was extremely dull inside, and he couldn't see anything. All of a sudden, two eyes got him in their glare, and the octopus rose up out of the murkiness. "I have been sitting tight for you!" said the octopus with a profound voice. "The waves have revealed to me your story. My recommendation is that give a sparkling scale to every last one of the other fish. You'll never again be the most wonderful fish in the sea, yet you'll discover how to be upbeat!" "I can't," the Rainbow Fish started to state, yet the octopus had just vanished into a foreboding shadow of ink. "Part with my scales? My lovely sparkling scales? Never! How might I be able to ever be cheerful without them," the Rainbow Fish thought.

All of a sudden, he felt a light dash of a balance. The little blue fish was back. He stated, "Rainbow Fish, kindly don't be furious. I simply need one little scale!" The Rainbow Fish faltered. "Just a single incredibly little shimmery scale. All things considered, possibly I wouldn't miss only one," he thought.

Carefully, the Rainbow Fish hauled out the littlest scale and offered it to the little fish. "Many thanks!" the little blue fish percolated energetically as he took care of the gleaming scale among his blue ones. A somewhat particular inclination came over the Rainbow Fish. For quite a while, he viewed the little blue fish swim to and fro with his new scale sparkling in the water.

The little blue fish zoomed through the sea with his scale blazing, so it didn't take some time before the Rainbow Fish was encompassed by the other fish. Everybody needed a sparkling scale. What's more, the more he parted with, the more pleased he became. At the point when the water around him loaded up with glinting scales, he, finally, felt comfortable among the other fish.

At last, the Rainbow Fish had just one sparkling scale left. His most prized assets had been parted with, yet he was extremely cheerful. "Please, Rainbow Fish! Come and play with us!" they called. "Here I come," said the Rainbow Fish and glad as a sprinkle, he swam off to join his companions.

14. The desolate starfish

Once Upon A Time.....

In a shielded pool of water, in the midst of the stones at the sea's edge, there carried on a little starfish named Stanley. The water was in every case, warm and salty where Stanley lived, and his homemade him exceptionally upbeat.

During the day, Stanley played in the sand that sparkled and shone in the warm daylight. Around evening time, after the sun slipped over the skyline, Stanley would cuddle up beside his preferred stone and fall fast asleep.

At that point, one day, Stanley saw that in spite of the fact that his house was comfortable, there was something missing.

It hushed up. Excessively calm.

There was never anybody to converse with. There was never anybody to play with. The little starfish acknowledged he was forlorn.

Stanley considered this throughout the day. At the point when the sun sneaked away that night, he was lonelier than he had ever been previously.

He moved over to his preferred stone and attempted to cuddle down to sleep, yet for reasons unknown, the stone presently appeared to be excessively hard and excessively cold.

"On the off chance that I simply had somebody to converse with," Stanley said to himself. "At that point, I wouldn't be forlorn."

Stanley gazed upward and started to watch the night sky. Individually, splendid, twinkling stars showed up, carrying delicate light to the dimness.

Stanley had never observed the stars. Hc was normally solid asleep before the moon laid its way over the water. This new sight was astonishing.

"That is it!" Stanley stated, sitting straight up.

"Why, I don't have a place in this little pool by any means. No big surprise, I'm so desolate. I should be a star that tumbled from the sky!"

"In any case, by what method will I ever get back up there?"

He could see the way the moon spread over the extraordinary sea, and he concluded that it must be the way back to the sky. He would simply need to figure out how to that way.

Throughout the night, Stanley lay alert, thinking about how he could get to that splendid moon way. Stanley had never left his comfortable minimal home. At last, he concluded that he would, in one way or another, need to go out into the extraordinary sea to discover the way to the stars in the sky.

At the point when the tide came in the following morning, Stanley crawled his way into the whirling water. The extraordinary waves immediately surged him away out into the incredible sea.

Stanley rolled and tumbled along these lines, and that in the forceful waves and the excursion about blew his mind. At last, the whirling and turning at long last halted, and Stanley floated gradually down to the sea depths'.

Here the water was not in any way decent and warm like his little pool. It was dull, cold, and baffling.

Simply then, a school of fish encompassed him. Stanley imagined this would be a decent time to get some information about the moon's way. Be that as it may, the fish just overlooked him and his inquiries, and swam away.

An old sea horse viewing from close by started to laugh.

"Senseless little starfish!" he giggled.

"The fish learn in school never to converse with outsiders. In the event that you need to think about the moon's way, I will disclose to you this; you will just discover it around evening time."

This baffled Stanley, yet he realized it must be valid, in light of the fact that he had never observed the moon's way during the day. Stanley chose to settle down in the sand and trust that night will come. He could utilize a rest after his sleepless night.

Stanley couldn't help thinking that he had just barely rested off when he heard an unusual clamor that sounded particularly like someone yelling.

WAKE UP!

Stanley opened his eyes. A tremendous hungry monster was swimming right toward him, licking its lips and smiling. Rapidly Stanley dodged into a major dull space under a stone, and crouched there, shaking with fear.

At the point when a voice talked from behind him, he was frightened to such an extent that he hopped straight up and knocked his head on the stone.

"It's alright at this point! Quiet down," the voice said. "That enormous puffer fish must have truly scared you! Golly, don't you realize a starfish ought to never rest out in the open that way? You were horrendously fortunate, you know! You nearly wound up as that large fish's supper! "

Stanley moved in the direction of the voice and got himself up close and personal with a quite little starfish.

"Goodness, thank you for sparing my life," Stanley heaved. "I had no clue it could be so hazardous over here!".

And afterward, Stanley flickered as he took a gander at the other little starfish. "Who are you? What's your name? Did you tumble from the sky, as well?" Stanley asked energetically. "Perhaps we can discover our way back together!"

The new little starfish laughed, "My name is Marcie. Tumble from the sky?? What on the planet would you say you are discussing?

So Stanley acquainted himself with Marcie and clarified how forlorn his little pool in the stones was, with nobody around to converse with or play with. He disclosed to her how he had seen the sky so loaded with stars and was searching for the moon's way to lead him up to his twinkling family in the sky.

"Gracious, Stanley!" Marcie chuckled. " You don't have a place up in the sky! You're a starfish, much the same as me! Starfish have a place in the water! Anyway, I'm apprehensive the moon's way could never lead you to the sky. The seahorse disclosed to me it's only an impression of the moon on the water."

Stanley took a gander at Marcie. "At that point, I surmise I ought to return home," he stated, "however it was so forlorn there."

At that point, Stanley started to educate his new companion concerning his peaceful, safe home, the warm sun, sparkling sand, and his preferred stone.

"That sounds awesome!" shouted Marcie. "Yet, why could possibly do you leave it? The sea is brimming with such huge numbers of threats, and the sun scarcely ever arrives at the profound waters."

"You're correct," murmured Stanley. "I would prefer truly not to remain around here. It's excessively cold, and hazardous. It's simply that I was so forlorn back there without anyone else's input."

"I have an awesome thought!" said Marcie. "In the event that you like, I'll return to the stones by the shore with you. I will remain and be your companion for consistently. We can talk and play together, and you will never be desolate again!"

"Will you? Truly? I might want that a ton, Marcie!" Stanley shouted joyfully. "We'll be closest companions! In any case, it will be elevated tide soon, so we would do well to hustle just a bit if we need to return home!"

So together, Marcie and Stanley moved along toward the sea's base, to where the swirling waters of the tide could convey them closer to shore.

They remained near together so that in the difficult situations, they wouldn't lose one another, and soon they tumbled securely once again into Stanley's shielded little pool in the midst of the stones at the water's edge.

Stanley gladly demonstrated Marcie around his comfortable minimal home. At that point, as the sun slipped over the skyline and the stars above started to fill the sky with twinkling brilliance, Stanley and Marcie cuddled up to Stanley's preferred stone, and the two of them fell fast asleep.

15. The Dinosaur Camping

There were four dinosaur companions who wanted to do everything together. They made fortifications, they swam in streams, and they played tag. What they had never done was to go outdoors.

One day Stegs chose to change that, so he said to his dinosaur companions: "We have to go outdoors under the stars. We can have a fire and eat sausages."

"I love eating hounds," Terry stated, however, no one listened on the grounds that Terry consistently discussed eating hounds. The remainder of the companions just gestured in understanding.

So the following day, they stuffed their tent and strolled to a close-by forest. They set up their tent on a level spot of grass around of pine trees.

"The branches are high to the point that we can positively cook franks securely," Bron said to his companions.

"I love eating hounds," Terry said.

The remainder of the companions accumulated wood and set up the tent. At that point, they strolled for 10 minutes and found a brook where they played catch and swam on their backs. Bron, Stegs, and Tri ate the plants from the base of the freshwater stream.

"Would we be able to eat hounds now?" Terry inquired. What's more, the time had come to return to the tent since it was getting dull, and they were in a new spot at the point when they kicked back they off a fire.

"Terry, don't contact the franks," Bron said. "We will do the cooking." And cook they did. They cooked 20 bundles of franks over the fire.

"We each have four bundles to eat," Stegs clarified.

"Would I be able to have 20?" Terry inquired.

"No!" They all replied.

So they each had four bundles as they discussed how much fun it was to camp. Following an hour of eating, the ball was in Tri's court to pose an inquiry.

"Where is the washroom? We did all eat four bundles of sausages, and I can't be the one in particular who needs to utilize one."

By the looks on his companions' faces, he was not alone.

"I don't accept we brought one," Bron conceded. "I don't figure it would have fit in the tent regardless of whether we'd have brought one."

Apparently, out of the blue, a young lady showed up.

"Greetings dinosaurs, my name is Leah, and I know where there is a potty you can pee on."

"I'm sorry, Leah, we have to do the other thing," Terry said.

"This is a potty you can pee and crap on. Tail me, and it's up a lot of blue advances."

Every one of the dinosaurs, with the exception of Stegs who expected to watch the fire, pursued Leah. It wasn't some time before they found the blue advances that prompted what Leah continued calling the Pee Fort. They all alternated, and even Stegs got a go-to go. At that point, they returned to their open-air fire and bid farewell to Leah, being certain to express gratitude toward her for the Pee Fort.

"That is the last time we go outdoors without pressing our potty," Tri reported before getting up to hit the sack.

"I love eating hounds," Terry said on the sign.

"We know. Goodbye."

16. The Unhappy Big Fish

This is one of the amazing bedtime stories for multi-year olds. In a puddle, almost a major stream carried on a gathering of fish. They all were companions and played with one another and were extremely cheerful. Among them, they carried on a greater fish. He was exceptionally pleased. Since he was greater, he thought of himself is a higher priority than the various fish. He was continually murmuring and protesting in the organization of the little fish.

Along these lines, at some point, one of the little fish let him know, "This puddle is unreasonably little for you. I'm amazed that you don't go to live in an enormous stream. There you would have many preferable buddies over little fish like us." The enormous fish considered those words, and undoubtedly, he imagined that it would be a smart thought for him to go to the huge waterway.

"I'm sick of these little fish," he pondered internally. "At the point when the winter comes, I'll have the option to leave this puddle and proceed to live in a major puddle where I can associate with increasingly recognized fish such as myself!"

Before long, the winter came and overflowed the puddle. Presently, the enormous fish could without much of a stretch swim to the large waterway. Everything was so large there, even the fish. He was resting close to a submerged cavern when he felt a solid present, and four enormous fish passed by pushing him aside. "Move away little fish," they said. "Don't you realize this cavern is held for large fish like us!"

"Little fish!" he thought. He had never been called that. Life in the waterway was totally different from the one in his puddle. He chose to cover up in some green growth and attempt to rest. Not long after, however, two tremendous and fearsome fish discovered him and started to assault him. He got away by swimming into somewhat split in a stone where they couldn't fit. He remained there for quite a while, trusting that the other fish will leave.

"Was this the manner in which life was in the waterway?" he thought. "Were these the upsides of living among the enormous fish?" He understood he had committed an error. Thus, he chose to come back to his puddle.

The voyage wasn't simple. He needed to swim upstream and be amazingly careful not to be assaulted by the other fish. At long last, following a few days, he arrived at his puddle and how euphoric and eased he felt. There was no other spot on the planet where he could rather be.

The adventure had made the huge fish a superior fish. He turned into the best of companions to the various little fish. He never protested again. Additionally, he was constantly prepared to disclose to them stories about the huge stream and the world past. The little fish were constantly glad to tune in.

17. The Tale Of Three Fishes

This is extraordinary compared to other short stories of Panchatantra in English with pictures for kids. Quite a long time ago, there lived three fishes in a delightful lake which was in a very heart of a thick forest. If the three fishes were firm companions and hung out. Every way altogether different from the other. The principal fish was insightful, and he generally made the wisest decision. If, at any point, some other animals in a difficult situation, they realized they could depend on him to enable them to out.

The subsequent fish was ingenious. If he was not the most astute of the animals in the lake, he generally figured out how to think something up so as to get himself out of the chaos. The third fish was, nonetheless, rather silly. In spite of the fact that he, for the most part, had good intentions, he would wind up getting both himself and his companions into inconvenience.

At some point, as the insightful fish was sobbing about in the water, he heard some fishermen talking. He was interested to hear what they needed to state. Thus he swam as near them as he challenged. He heard the fishermen state that they would land there the following morning to fish in the lake. The shrewd fish immediately swam to where different fishes were and mentioned to them what he had heard. He additionally revealed to them that he had chosen to swim through channel and getaway.

The insightful fish asked, "Why not join me with the goal that we can reach securely!" The ingenious fish won't and stated, "This has been my home for such huge numbers of years. I can't leave it! I will remain and see what should be possible!" "you two stress excessively! Nothing will occur by any stretch of the imagination," the stupid fish said and swam away.

The fishermen came the following day and got numerous fishes. Among them were the creative fish and silly fish. The ingenious fish laid as yet professing to be dead and was put at the ground by the lake. He unobtrusively slipped go into the lake, and swam away. The absurd fish continued hurling about until one of the fishermen struck him hard and slaughtered him. A couple of days after the fact, the shrewd fish returned. He and the clever fish had understood that their companion was so silly. "In the event that he had thought carefully, he may have been with us still," they said.

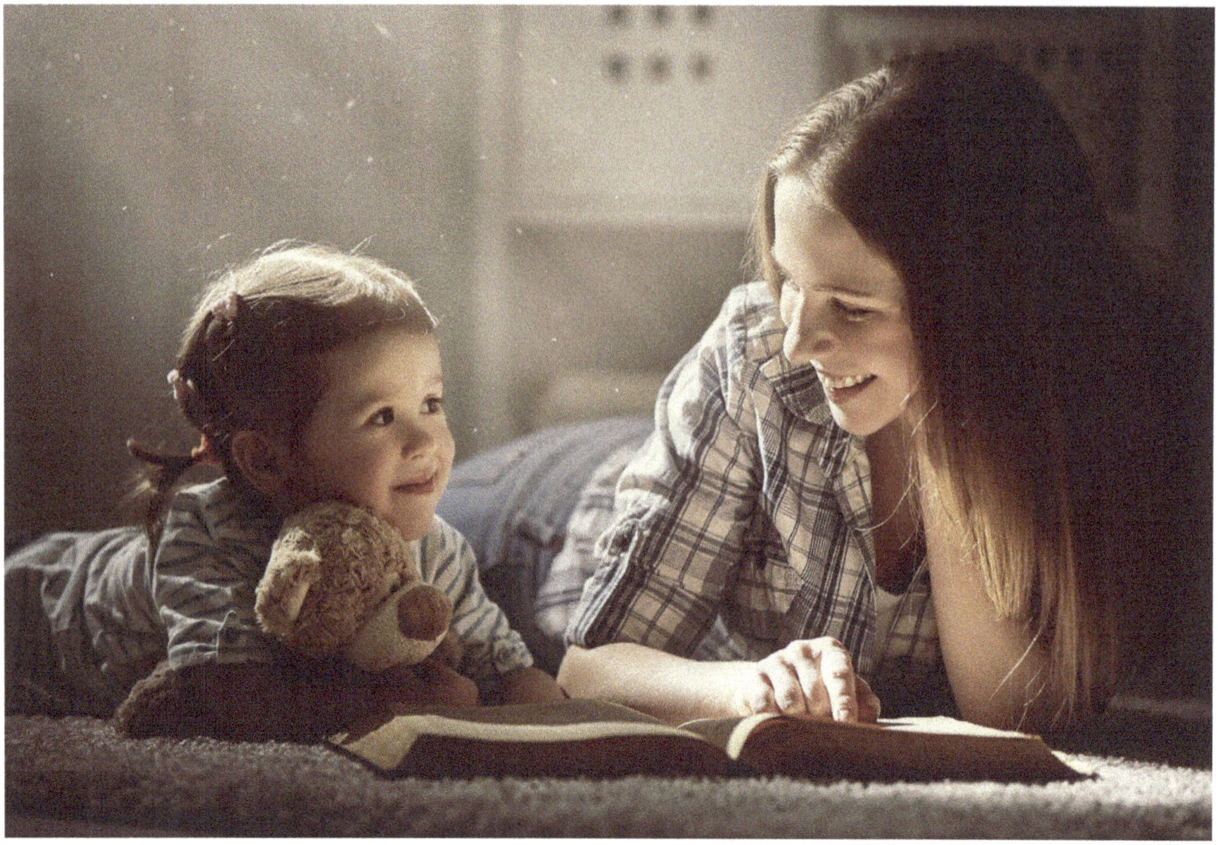

10 JUNGLE ANIMALS PROTAGONIST STORIES FOR CHILDREN BEDTIME

What Is A Jungle Bedtime Story?

Bedtime stories will be stories that are told after your child has gotten into bed for the night. Commonly they will request you to sit with them. This is a simple chance to offer to disclose to them a story. Young children particularly love this since it is a treat for them and makes them feel really important at that time.
You can either peruse an exemplary story from a book, locate a speedy one on the web, or let one know from memory. Oftentimes an incredible bedtime story is ad-libbed to suit the state of mind of your child in that specific minute. These stories are ordinary ones that have been told for a long time from multiple points of view. Well, known stories incorporate ones about princesses and sovereigns, incredible monsters and knights, children on undertakings, and energizing tales with no specific consummation of them. This last sort of story is intriguing in light of the fact that it enables you to draw a similar story out over numerous evenings to keep your child intrigued and continually needing more.

Create Memories Together

Perusing a bedtime story to your children is an incredible method to associate with them. It gets the family closer to a private setting that additionally makes the child feel extraordinary. Recollections are made as stories are told. Your child will anticipate you sitting with them before they float off to sleep. This time together is something that they will consistently value. These valuable minutes advantage everybody included, and you will find that you anticipate the bedtime stories nearly to such an extent or more than your little one.

Benefits Of Bedtime Stories

Recounting to bedtime stories is gainful. Your child will discover sleep arriving in a quiet manner with an extraordinary story in their ears. It connects with their creative mind while giving them great dream material, and has been appeared to quiet down a bustling child. Children do will, in general, be animated now and again, particularly around evening time, and a decent story will put their feelings of trepidation to rest and permit them much-required relaxation. You can make a story that gives them that the monster under their bed isn't so terrible, or that the shadows on their divider are their companions. The conceivable outcomes are unfathomable with inventive answers for any nighttime issue.

Bedtime stories additionally show your child in manners that are like tales, legends, and fairy tales. Perusing bedtime stories is a convincing method for helping your child develop into a well-molded person. The fun part about bedtime stories is that you can make one up yourself and art it into something one of a kind and uncommon. An exceptional story goes far for a child with open ears, and you will end up being a wellspring of extraordinary enthusiasm for your children.

A complete rundown of jungle animals would take you weeks and weeks to peruse since there are a huge number of animals living on the planet's jungles, otherwise called tropical rainforests. About portion of all the animal species on earth—warm-blooded creatures, flying creatures, creepy crawlies, creatures of land and water, and reptiles—would be on that rundown of jungle animals.

Moreover, the world contains a wide range of jungles or downpour forests, and the rundown of jungle animals would be diverse for every jungle.

If we can make a short rundown of the absolute most fascinating jungle animals with regards to every one of the downpour forests around the planet. We can have a rundown of jungle animals for every jungle that incorporates a top predator or two, a couple of the biggest animals in that jungle, a few primates, at least one reptiles, and a few flying creatures.

Here Are Our Lists Of Jungle Animals

Rundown Of Jungle Animals In The Amazon

Top Predators: Jaguars, Cougars, Ocelots

Biggest Animal: The Tapir

Rat: Capybara (The World's Largest Rodent!)

Reptiles: Anaconda, Bushmaster (harmful snake) and Caimans (a few species; the biggest is the dark caiman)

Creatures of land and water: Poison Dart Frogs

Winged animals: Harpy Eagle, Macaws (counting the red macaw and the hyacinth macaw)

Primates: Spider monkeys, howler monkeys, capuchin monkeys, squirrel monkeys

Fish: Piranha

Bug: Leaf-Cutter Ant

Rundown Of Jungle Animals In Africa

Top Predator: The Leopard

Huge Animals: The Jungle Elephant, The Okapi

Reptiles: Rock Python, Nile Crocodile, Mambas (a few types of harmful snakes)

Fowls: Gray Parrot, Crowned Eagle

Primates: Chimpanzees, Bonobos, Gorillas, Mandrills, Baboons, Colobus Monkeys, Bush Babies

Fish: Tiger Fish

Creepy crawly: Termite

Rundown of Jungle Animals In Asia

Top Predators: The Tiger, The Leopard

Bears: Sun Bear, Sloth Bear

Bat: Flying Fox (Fruit-Eating Bat)

Biggest Animals: Sumatran Rhinoceros, Elephant, Water Buffalo

Fowls: Cockatoo, Black Eagle

Reptiles: Saltwater Crocodile, Burmese Python, Cobra (a few species)

Primates: Orangutan, Gibbons, Macaque Monkeys, Langur Monkeys, Tarsiers

Fish: Betta (Siamese fighting fish)

1. Baby Bubba goes to the Jungle

Once there was a little baby kid called Bubba. Bubba had splendid blue eyes and brilliant twists, and everybody who saw him adored him immediately. He had a caretaker called Jiji who had cared for him as far back as he was a serious little baby, and she was partial to him.

The Army Officer was Budda's father, and they lived in a delightful white house on the Hills. Around the house was a nursery, and outside the nursery, there was a jungle for miles and miles, and a wide range of winged creatures and animals lived in the jungle.

Little Bubba preferred playing on the yard with his pets, Miow, the feline, and Wooff-Wooff, the canine, and the two of them adored him profoundly. Miow-Miow never scratched him, and Wooff-Wooff remained on his two rear legs to perform interesting stunts to make Bubba chuckle.

Each morning after breakfast, Bubba tossed bread pieces to the little winged animals in the yard. The winged creatures sat in the trees and hung tight for him, and sang about him till he left the house. Bubba wanted to sustain them and play with them. Miow-Miow watched the winged creatures. However, she never attempted to get them since she realized that Bubba adored them.

Be that as it may, one day, when Bubba was nourishing the feathered creatures, a major snake called Hoody, who lived in the nursery, came crawling up close to the veranda. He attempted to get a portion of the flying creatures while they were eating. However, Bubba saw him and got out, "Leave, awful, Hoody, leave!"

Bubba's caretaker listened to him and came hurrying to perceive what the issue was. Seeing her, Hoody slithered away into his opening under a major tree in the nursery.

Presently Hoody was a shrewd snake and was consistently up to some devilishness. Hoody figured it is enjoyable to take bubba out of the jungle, where all other wild animals are living.

One day, he found himself in the jungle to see an old companion of his, Tig, the Tiger, and talk the issue over with him. Hoody inquired as to whether he might want to meet a little baby kid, and Tig licked his lips and stated, "H'M! we should see."

At that point, Hoody went further into the jungle and met Prowl, the Wolf. "How might you want to meet a little baby?" asked Hoody, and Prowl, the Wolf, licked his lips and stated, "aha!" and that's it.

Somewhat further on Hoody met Bluf, the large dark-colored Bear,then he asked him a question that "what will you do if you saw a little baby in the jungle. What's more, Bluf stood up on his rear legs and stated, Oh! It would be pleasant, exceptionally decent, to be sure!"

And afterward, Poonda, the enormous wild Elephant, came pulverizing through the jungle, and Hoody immediately hurried out of his way. "How might you want to meet a little .. " he shouted out, yet Poonda made a boisterous commotion with his trunk and ran on. All things considered, Hoody was fulfilled, and he snickered, thinking Poonda may stomp on Bubba when he goes to the jungle.

After this, Hoody returned home to his gap under the tree in Bubba's nursery and watched and paused. At some point, when Wooff-Wooff had headed out to pursue a wild bunny, Meow-Meow was fast asleep in the sun.

Hoody slid out of his opening rapidly and drew close to Bubba, waving his head to and fro, and shooting out his little tongue, while the sun shone on his smooth sparkling skin. Gracious, pretty Hoody!" said Bubba, "you're devious. Leave!" "No," said Hoody sweetly, "I'm not devious, dear Bubba, and I realize where some wonderful blossoms develop. Accompany me, and I'll show you!" "No," said Bubba, shaking his head.

However, Hoody kept on taking a gander at him consistently, and soon Bubba slid down from the verandah and drew close to him. At that point, Hoody chuckled and moved back rapidly into the thick piece of the nursery, and Bubba pursued him.

At the point when the Nanny came back to the porch with Bubba's Noah's Ark, and she saw his little vacant seat and Miow-Miow asleep in the sun, she was frightened and went around calling

Bubba's name. At that point, Bubba's Mommy turned out, and afterward, his Daddy, and they searched the nursery for quite a while, yet couldn't discover any hint of him.
At that point, Miow-Miow woke up, and Wooff-Wooff returned, and the two of them thought about what was happening. Before long, some little flying creatures overhead shouted to them to stand out for them. They stated, "Bubba pursued Hoody, the Snake, into the jungle, and he will be lost and hurt by the wild animals except if he is brought back. Brisk! Fast! Follow him!"
Thus Wooff-Wooff raced to Bubba's Father and Mother and attempted to let them know. He ran in reverse and advances attempting to highlight the jungle, and yapped and woofed. At that point, woof-woof set out to the jungle to discover Bubba, and Bubba's folks pursued.

Presently after Bubba had pursued Hoody a little route through the nursery, the snake went to a little way, which prompted a wrecked piece of the nursery divider. "You should creep through here," said Hoody, "the pretty blossoms are on the opposite side." So Bubba slithered through and wound up in the jungle.

Further on! further on!" cried Hoody, each time Bubba halted to assemble any, "there are prettier ones further on." And so Bubba continued forever till he came to where Tig the Tiger lay asleep in the long grass. "Presently's your time," murmured Hoody in his ear, "here's the little baby I outlined for you." And Tig jumped up with thunder.
In any case, Bubba was anything but somewhat scared, and he just snickered and said, "what a major, huge Miow-Miow!" He settled his head in his delicate hide, and Tig enjoyed it so much, he murmured with enchanting simply like Miow-Miow did when she was satisfied. Hoody resented this, and seeing that Bubba befriended Tig, he called to Bubba, "Come, how about we proceed to discover more blooms."
Also, Bubba kissed Tig farewell, and pursued Hoody further into the jungle, till they met Prowl, the Wolf. "Here's the little baby," murmured Hoody. Furthermore, Prowl stated, "Ha!" and was going to spring upon him. However, Bubba just snickered and stated, "What a major Wooff-Wooff!" and congratulated him on the head, and investigated his eyes. Slink then licked Bubba's hands and searched around him simply like Wooff-Wooff.
This is senseless," said Hoody furiously. "Come now, it is practically nightfall, and we should return home," and he drove the best approach to where Bluf, the huge dark colored Bear, lived.
Furthermore, Bluf stated, "Gracious! Exceptionally pleasant, decent to be sure!" And got Bubba up in his arms and embraced him. "Much the same as my Nanny does!" snickered Bubba, and he tapped Bluf's cheeks and kissed him, and Bluf embraced him more to keep him warm.

Only then, there was a boisterous trumpeting commotion, and Bluf put Bubba down on the ground, and Hoody slid off into the grass, murmuring. "Presently, Poonda is coming!"

In any case, when Poonda came and saw the little baby Bubba, he recollected that he had not generally been a wild elephant, however, had once had a place with a pleasant man.

What's more, Bubba's Father discovered him after he pursued woof-woof into the jungle. Wooff-Wooff followed the young man by his aroma and discovered him riding on Poonda's back. At that point, Poonda let Bubba's Father sit on his back as well. Thus they returned in triumph with Bubba and his Father on Poonda's back and great Wooff-Wooff yapping and searching close by. The underhanded snake Hoody went into the jungle and never attempted to trouble Bubba until the end of time.

2. Monster in the Jungle

Monster in the Jungle

Sometime in the past, a savvy lion lived in the jungle. He was constantly regarded for his knowledge and graciousness. Every one of the animals used to go to him to examine their issues.

A couple of miles from the jungle, there was an unfilled cavern. Every one of the animals realized it was betrayed, and nobody lived there. Be that as it may, one day, they saw a monster entering the cavern. The monster was malicious and needed to eat the animals; however, no one would converse with him. He decide to welcome every one of the animals to the cavern for a gathering and later eat them. He knew the lord of the jungle was savvy, and he would not enable any animal to go to the gathering, so he did nOt welcome him. He additionally realized how fearless and solid the lion was, so he was truly scared of him.

Every one of the animals prepared for the gathering and assembled at a spot to go to the cavern. In any case, Zebra called the attention to the King of the Jungle was missing, thereby they all plead to the lion to request that he go with them. The lion saw every one of the animals together and asked them where they were going. At the point when they educated him regarding the gathering, he quickly comprehended the monster's arrangement, so he advised every one of the animals to hold up here, and he went to the cavern alone. Seeing the lion, the monster got truly scared and attempted to run; however, the lion got him. The monster requested absolution; however, the lion just pardoned him depending on the prerequisite that he would leave the buckle and never return. Thus, the monster concurred and left.

All the animals expressed gratitude toward the lion for sparing them from the monster and lived joyfully together.

2. A Dance in the Forest with the Parrot

In a major forest, there lived numerous animals and winged animals. One day a portion of the feathered creatures were discourse about the manner in which the animals live. The parrot stated, "Take a gander at me. I don't eat any fledgling or animal I simply like foods grown from the ground them constantly. I despise taking a gander at these animals as they chase different animals and eat them". I feel that we the winged creatures are the best in the forest as we don't eat different flying creatures for our endurance".
Numerous winged creatures consented to this contention and portrayed their very own feelings:

The sparrow stated: I eat the little bugs that make mischief to others that don't imply that I resemble these animals who execute all other great animals.

The woodpecker stated: See, I ensure trees by eating the white ants under their bark. In the event that I don't do such a large number of trees would have been destroyed by these white ants and different creepy crawlies.

The weaver winged animal: You know that I am the best in the forest in making the home. Show me any animal that can do like me. These animals are lethargic and live like shakes in all seasons.

The murmuring winged animal stated: I drink the nectar from the blossoms and keeping in mind that doing so, I don't hurt the blooms. In the event that helps in fertilization and make the forest look bright with numerous blossoms.
In this manner, numerous flying creatures portrayed their own stories and methods for living. In the interim, they saw a group of elephants going under the trees. The parrot shouted at them: Hey, large beasts, do you realize that feathered creatures are the best ones in the forest. You animals wreck forest, eat different animals, and make carnage for your endurance.

One of the elephants reacted by saying: I don't have the foggiest idea what you are talking. However, I can advise this to different animals as I will go to the gathering called by the Lion.

The Lion – the ruler of the forest – is perched on a major stone encompassed by numerous animals. The gathering started with the point, "In what manner will we praise the beginning of dash." At that point, the elephant interceded and stated: we feel that we are extraordinary in the forest. I heard a parrot saying that the winged creatures are the best since they don't eat different flying creatures for their very own endurance. Lets initially take care of this issue, and by concluding who is the best in the forest, the feathered creatures are we the animals.

Every one of the animals got bothered at the announcement of the parrot shared by the elephant. The wolf stated: Let's call the flying creatures here, and we as a whole can murder them and eat them immediately, then there is no issue. Haa Haaa joined different animals.

Chill off: said the Lion. On the off chance that the flying creatures feel that they are the best in the forest, we will enable them to demonstrate. They said that they don't eat different flying creatures; however, it is bogus. They do eat different winged animals for their endurance. You know that the hawks are consistently watchful for chicks of hens and peahens. They eat cruelly every one of the chicks. Feathered creatures are fools and unable animals. I feel sorry for them. Let's play with them for quite a while and demonstrate our strength. Dear fox, call every one of the fowls without a moment's delay here.

The fox moved toward the mangrove and shouted at the winged creatures. You appear to have an inclination that you are the best in the forest. Lets us demonstrate who is best in the forest. Every one of you can go to our gathering place close to the lake and substantiate yourselves.

Hearing this, the winged animals felt tested. Every one of them flew towards the gathering place.

In the gathering place, the most warmed contentions occurred.

Seeing the warmth produced, the Lion said. The meeting is suspended to tomorrow toward the beginning of the day and asked every one of the animals and winged creatures to dispense.

At night the terrific elderly person who regularly visits forest and helps animals and winged creatures by treating them went to the gathering place and solicited some from the fowls as yet staying there: I heard a disturbance toward the evening what befell all of you. I heard the boisterous hints of animals and feathered creatures as well. Do you have any issues, and would I be able to be of any assistance to you?

The feathered creatures stated: we had issued to comprehend between the fowls and the animals. We will demonstrate who is the best in the forest. We contend we are the best, yet they contend as barbarously as they can for their predominance. It is great that you have come. Why not desire the gathering tomorrow and help us.

The fabulous elderly person said Ok, I would come tomorrow.

The following day every morning, every one of the fowls and the animals assembled at the gathering place — the excellent elderly person set aside some effort to show up. His appearance was invited by the Lion, who was once spare by the fantastic elderly person. The dear fantastic elderly person, I am happy that you are here, hear every one of our contentions, and reveal to us who is the best in the forest.

Both the sides adequately advised the great elderly person. The feathered creatures and the animals got quiet and anticipated the judgment of the fantastic elderly person.
The great elderly person stated: The contention of the feathered creatures that they don't eat different winged animals is both wrong and compose. So in the contentions, the feathered creatures and the animals both win and lose. That makes the issue nil. The winged creatures and animals got confounded at this. Seeing their faces, especially of the Lion's the stupendous elderly person explained it further:

In spite of the fact that the hens and pen hens go under the group of flying creatures, they generally live on the ground, and they don't fly for their endurance. They run for their endurance, so really go under the group of animals. The chicks of the winged creatures additionally don't fly; they simply run on the ground, so they are likewise animals. Since Eagles eat these chicks, it adds up to eating different feathered creatures for their endurance as the animals do. Which means winged animals eat and don't eat different feathered creatures for their endurance.

The most important thing is this: If animals like Lion, tiger, cheetah, fox, and wolf don't eat different animals like sheep, goat, and so forth, the number of inhabitants in these grass-eating animals increment making the forest dry and hard for all to endure. Likewise, the winged animals help in fertilization and cross-fertilization, engendering of trees, and help add excellence to the forest. The forest gets dull, with no one of you. So neither the winged creatures nor the animals are best in the forest, the forest itself is the best since it gives us nourishment, safe house, and insurance from the individuals.

Hearing this, the Lion stated: what a splendid man are you, my dear great elderly person. I concur with you that the forest is the best. The flying creatures do twittered a similar sentiment.

At that point, the squirrel stated: this is the best time to commend the beginning of spring. Let's move... .

Every one of the animals moved and made joyfully... .

3. The Clever Monkey

This is an astounding jungle story for kids. Once, quite a while in the past in the jungle, the animals were assembled around the watering opening. They were pitiful on the grounds that another lion had come to live in their piece of the jungle. This lion was an awful harasser. He tied the elephant's trunk in a tangle and put natural products on rhino's horn. The lion even played draw an obvious conclusion with giraffe's spots and made interesting pictures.

The animals met to perceive how they could dispose of the lion. Above them on a tree, a monkey was tuning in. He started chuckling. "For what reason are you giggling?" asked the animals. "I am chuckling in light of the fact that all of you are scared of the lion. I am not scared of him. He has been working for me for quite a long time," said the monkey.

This idea of the monkey making the lion work for him made the animals snicker. The lion approached the animals and thundered, "For what reason are you chuckling?" The animals mentioned to the lion what the monkey had said. "Where is that monkey?" asked the lion. The animals highlighted the tree where the monkey had been sitting, yet he was no more.

The lion raged off to discover the monkey. Far away from the watering gap, the monkey was sitting in the way. When the lion saw the monkey, he approached him and snarled, "The animals revealed to me that you said you were not terrified of me and that I worked for you!" "That isn't what I let them know, companion! I disclosed to them I fear you and that I wish that I could work for you," answered the monkey.

"Please, lion! We should go see those senseless animals and ensure they know the reality," said the monkey. Together, they started down the way toward the watering opening. They had possibly gone a couple of steps down the way when the monkey grabbed his leg and cried.

"What's going on with you?" snarled the lion. "I stepped on a sharp stone. I am anxious about the possibility that I can't stroll back with you," said the monkey. "You need to tell every one of the animals that you truly fear me," said the lion. "All things considered, I could make it in the event that you would let me ride on your back," said the monkey. The lion concurred, and the monkey jumped on the lion's back and started strolling down the way.

They had possibly gone a couple of steps when the monkey shouted out. "What's up?" asked the lion. "I'm making some hard memories sitting on your back. It is exceptionally knotty! It might be ideal if that I had a seat," said the monkey. The lion helped the monkey make a seat out of palm leaves. The monkey sat on the seat and stated, "This is greatly improved! How about we go!"

They had possibly gone a couple of steps when the monkey shouted out. "What's going on?" snarled the lion. "I'm apprehensive about dropping out of the seat. It might be ideal in the event that I had something to hold," cried the monkey. The lion helped the monkey tie a few wines around his neck. "This is vastly improved! How about we go," said the monkey.

They had gone a couple of more advances when the monkey again shouted out. "What is it presently?" said the lion. "There is a lot of flies around here. I need something to swat them away," said the monkey. The lion got an enormous verdant branch and offered it to the monkey. "Much obliged to you, lion! This will help," said the lion. "How about we go!"

As the monkey and the lion drew near to the watering gap, the monkey sat up high in the seat, grabbed the vines, swatted the lion with the verdant, and shouted, "Better believe it!" The lion was shocked to the point that he ran fast. He ran so fast that he ran directly past the watering opening where every one of the animals was assembled. "Please, you sluggish lion, it's no time to rest!" shouted the monkey.

Every one of the animals started to snicker as they saw the monkey on the lion's back. As they went past the watering gap, the monkey swung off the lion's back and into the trees. The giggling of the animals rang in the lion's ears as he ran down the way. He never returned to that piece of the jungle. He may, in any case, be running, and the shrewd monkey may even now be snickering.

4. The Wolf And The Seven Young Goslings

Quite a long time ago,

There was, at one time, an old goose who had seven young goslings and adored them as just a mother can cherish her children. When she was going into the wood to look for provender, and before setting off she called every one of the seven to her and stated, "Dear children, I am obliged to go into the wood, so be wary against the wolf; for in the event that he gets in here he will gobble you up, plumes, skin, whatnot. The reprobate regularly masks himself, yet you can without much of a stretch, remember him by his harsh voice and dark paws."

The children replied, "Dear mother, we will take extraordinary care; you may abandon any anxiety." So the old woman supported and set off brightly for the wood.

After a short time, somebody thumped at the entryway, and cried, "Open, open, my dear children; your mom is here, and has brought something for every one of you."

In any case, the goslings before long apparent, by the unpleasant voice, that it was the wolf. "We won't open," said they; "you are not our mom, for she has a sweet and beautiful voice; however, your voice is unpleasant – you are the wolf."

Immediately the wolf set off to a vendor and purchased an enormous chunk of chalkt. Back he came, thumped at the entryway, and cried, "Open, open, my dear children; your mom is here, and has brought something for every one of you."

Yet, the wolf had laid his dark paw on the window-ledge, and when the children saw it, they cried, "We won't open; our mom has not dark feet like you – you are the wolf."

So the wolf ran off to the bread cook, and stated, "I have harmed my foot, put some mixture on it." And when the pastry specialist had put it with batter, the wolf went to the mill operator and cried, "Strew some supper on my paws." But the mill operator contemplated internally, "The wolf needs to trick somebody," and he dithered to do it; till the wolf stated, "On the off chance that you don't do it on the double, I will gobble you up." So the mill operator was apprehensive and made his paws white. Such is the method for the world!

Presently returned the maverick for the third time, thumped, and stated, "Open the entryway, dear children; your mom has gotten back home and has brought something for every one of you out of the wood."

Goslings cried, saying "Show us your paws first, that we may see whether you are, without a doubt, our mom." So he laid his paws on the window-ledge, and when the goslings saw that they were white, they trusted it was okay, and opened the entryway; and who should come in yet the wolf!

They shouted out and attempted to shroud themselves; one bounced under the table, another into the bed, the third into the broiler; the fourth ran into the kitchen, the fifth jumped into a chest, the 6th under the wash-tub, and the seventh got into the clock-case. Yet, the wolf held onto them and remained on no service with them; in a steady progression, he ate them all up, aside from the youngest, who is in the clock-case he couldn't discover. At the point when the wolf had eaten his fill, he walked forward, laid himself down in the green knoll under a tree, and then sleep.
The house-entryway stood all the way open; table, seats, seats, were all overthrown; the wash-tub lay in the remains; covers and pads were detached the bed. She searched for her children. However, no place might she be able to discover them; she considered them each by name, yet no one replied. Finally, when she went to the youngest, a bit of squeaking voice replied, "Dear mother, I am in the clock-case." She hauled him out, and he disclosed to her how the wolf had come and had gobbled up all the others. You may think about how she sobbed for her dear children.
Finally, in her sorrow, she went out, and the youngest gosling ran adjacent to her. What's more, when she went to the knoll, there lay the wolf under the tree, wheezing till the limbs shook. She strolled around and inspected him on all sides, till she saw that something was moving and kicking about inside him.

"Would it be able to be," thought she, "that my poor children whom he has gulped for his dinner are yet alive?" So she sent the small gosling back to the house for scissors, needle, and string, and started to cut up the monster's stomach. Hardly had she given one cut, when out came the leader of a gosling, and when she had cut somewhat further, the six leaped out consistently, not having taken the least harmed, in light of the fact that the avaricious monster had gulped down them down. That was a delight! They grasped their mom softly and avoided about as exuberant as a tailor at his wedding.

In any case, the old goose stated, "Presently proceed to discover me six enormous stones, which we will put inside the insatiable beast while he is still fast asleep." The goslings got the stones in all flurry, and they put them inside the wolf; and the old goose closed him up again in an incredible rush, while he not even once moved nor took any notification.

Presently when the wolf finally woke up and got upon his legs, he discovered he was parched and wished to go to the spring to drink. Be that as it may, when he started to move the stones started to shake and shake inside him, till he cried, –

"What's this thundering and tumbling,

What's this shaking like the bones,

I had eaten six little geese,

However, they've turned out just stones."

Furthermore, when he went to the spring and bowed down his head to drink, the overwhelming stones overbalanced him, and he went head over heels. Presently when the seven goslings saw this, they came running up, crying boisterously, "The wolf is dead, the wolf is dead!" and moved for satisfaction all-round the spring and their mom with them.

5. A Life in the Woods

One day a deer was conceived. His name was Bambi. His mom washed him done with her tongue.

"Bambi," she said. "My little Bambi."

The young Bambi was interested in everything. He learned he was a deer, as was his mom.Other deer in the forest, and sometime he would meet them. He learned the path his mom pursued was made by the deer. Bugs and critters, sounds, and scents. Such huge numbers of marvels to investigate!

Sometimes on a path, all of a sudden, his mom would stop still. She would open her ears wide and tune in from all bearings. First-over there! At that point here! Bambi would pause. Finally, when she stated, "It's good. There's no threat. We can go," at that point, both of them would start on the path once more. However, he didn't have the foggiest idea why they needed it.

At some point, his mom took him to the glade just because. He started to head out to the open clearing; however, she bounced directly before him. "Stop!" said she. "Remain here. I should go out first. Hang tight till I call for you. Be I start to run, you should pivot and run over into the forested areas exceptionally fast. Try not to stop. Do you get me?"

Bambi's mom gradually ventured out beyond all detectable inhibitions knoll. She sniffed all around. She looked along these lines and that, alert and careful. After a moment, she stated, "It's fine, Bambi. Nothing to stress over. Please!" He limited out to meet her.

Goodness, what a brilliant sun! Back in the forested areas, Bambi had seen a stray sunbeam once in a while, however here, the splendid sweltering sun warmed him everywhere. He felt heavenly and bounced high into the air. Each time he arrived on grass milder than any grass he had ever felt. At that point, he jumped back up once more, over and over.

In certain spots, the blossoms were so thick, and they made a sweet floor covering. In any case, what was that minor thing moving noticeably all around? "See, Mother!" said Bambi. "The bloom is flying." Why that blossom probably expected to move such a lot, Bambi thought, that it severed right its stem to ascend and move noticeable all around.

"That is not a blossom, Bambi," said the mother, "it's a butterfly."

At that point – Thump, pound, pound! On a stone was a young bunny, a hare, pounding its foot.

"Hi, there!" grinned Hare, raising one tall ear. "Need to play?"

"Sure!" said Bambi.

"Catch me!" Hare bounced off the stone into the grass, jump jumping ceaselessly. Bambi was somewhat faster at running and bouncing, yet Hare was better at covering up, so both of them made some fine memories.

Over the blooms, a tall, fleecy, highly contrasting tail was sliding over to them. "Why I'd realize that tail anyplace!" said Hare. "It's my companion, Skunk. He's under the blossoms. Skunk?" And sufficiently sure, a high contrast head sprung up.

"This is Bambi," said Hare. Before long them, three were investigating the knoll, sniffing its rich, profound scents.

After temporarily, Hare and Skunk needed to return home. Bambi glanced around. "Mother! Where are you?" At the most distant side of the knoll, he saw her, with an animal that looked simply like her.

"come meet my sister Ena," said Bambi's mom. "Furthermore, her two minimal ones." Bambi bounced over. Two grovels, little Faline and her sibling Gobo, were running all through their mom's legs.

Faline gave a jump and landed directly before Bambi, at that point, hopped back to Gobo. With care, Bambi ventured up to her. Faline jumped off to the other side, and Gobo pursued. Before long them, three were pursuing each other here and there the grass.

"Presently run off and play, every one of you," said Bambi's mom.

Consistently from that point forward, the three young deer played and babbled. They hustled and pursued, they snacked numerous strawberries and blueberries on the shrubberies, and sometimes they just talked.

At some point, Bambi stated, "Do you realize what peril implies?"

"Something awful," murmured Gobo.

"Be that as it may, what is it?" said Bambi.

"I recognize what threat is," said Faline. "It's what you flee from." But soon, they were pursuing and playing once more.

Bambi's mom and Ena came up. "Please now," they said. "It's time to return home."

Far away at the highest point of a slope, two huge pleased deer came into see, with gigantic heads of horns.

Going to them, Faline stated, "Who are they?"

"Those are your dads," said Ena.

"In the event that you are savvy and don't run into potential harm," said Bambi's mom to her child, "sometime or another, you will grow up as large and attractive as your dad. What's more, you will have prongs, as well." Bambi's heart expands proudly.
As Bambi developed, he learned how to sniff the air. He could tell if his companion Hare was coming, or if a fox had recently jogged by. He could tell on the off chance that it would rain soon. One evening came a furious tempest. Lightning flashed, and thunder slammed. Bambi thought the apocalypse had come. In any case, when he lay by his mom's side, he had a sense of security.

One day when Bambi meandered about in the forested areas, he happened upon a sharp, horrendous smell. Inquisitive, he tailed it. It prompted a clearing, where stood a peculiar animal. He had never observed such an animal. It stood upon its back legs, and in its two arms, it held something long and dark – might it be able to be the third leg? The smell of the animal in some way or another filled him with fear. The animal raised its long dark arm. Instantly, Bambi's mom surged up to him.
"Run, Bambi, run! As fast as possible!"

Bambi's mom limited over bushes and shrubberies. He kept pace close to her till they were back at their verdant home.

Afterward, Bambi's mom stated, "Did you see the Human?" Bambi gestured, yes. "That is the person who brings threat," she said. Furthermore, two shivered.
Bambi was all the while developing. The first time he woke to discover his mom gone from his side, he was scared. It was early morning and still dim. "Mother! Mother!" he got out. A huge

shadow drew nearer, greater than his mother's. Remaining before a pool of evening glow, a Great Old Buck looked pleased and harsh.
The Buck said who are you calling with a grimace. "Wouldn't you be able to deal with yourself?" Bambi didn't set out an answer. He brought down his head in disgrace. "Gaze upward," said the Old Buck, "Hear me out. Watch. Smell. Discover for yourself. You will be fine without anyone else."

The leaves fell, and Bambi became considerably taller. His mom started disregarding him to an ever-increasing extent, letting him meet other deer and animals of the forest. Faline, Gobo, Hare, and Skunk were as yet Bambi's closest companions, yet he likewise found different animals intriguing to watch and sometimes amusing to play with.
One wet winter day, the horrible smell of Humans cleared over the forest. The fragrance was solid to such an extent that there must be numerous Humans in a gathering! Most animals immediately fled out of peril. In any case, some were not as fortunate. With the tracker's boisterous clamor and extraordinary force, numerous animals were executed, and one of them was Bambi's mom.

After that horrible day, Bambi felt lost. He meandered about. How could this horrendous thing have occurred? All of a sudden, the Great Old Buck ventured out before him.

"Were you out in the knoll when it occurred?" the Old Buck said.

"Truly," said Bambi.

"Furthermore, you do not require your mom?" said the Buck.

Abruptly Bambi felt loaded with fortitude. "I can deal with myself!" he stated, turning upward.

The Great Old Buck grinned. "Hear me out," he said. "Smell. Watch. Learn to live and be careful. Discover for yourself. Presently goodbye." And he disappeared into the profound forest.
Winter came. Solid and unpleasant virus twists moved through the forested areas. Profound snow covered the forest floor. There was little nourishment to eat. Bambi felt ravenous and cold constantly. Almost all the bark on the trees had been stripped away by hungry deer. All things considered, the virus wind rankled on, for quite a while.

Gobo had consistently been littler than Bambi and Feline. He shuddered constantly. He could barely stand up any longer.

One day a group of crows flew overhead, shouting noisily. "Caw! Caw!" The geese likewise shouted in the sky, "Stare! Ogle!" They cautioned of the Humans coming – once more!

Bunny bounced all over in alert. "We're encompassed! They are all over the place!" A solitary blast smashed like thunder, and one goose tumbled from the sky. Every one of the animals ran like distraught, even the little titmouse. Another short accident like thunder and a fox tumbled down on the forest floor. Blast! Blast!

Rabbit shouted to Bambi, "We need to leave!" Bambi and Hare started to bound away. In any case, was that Gobo, lying in the day off?

"Gobo!" said Bambi. "Where are your mom and Faline?"
"I tumbled down," said Gobo. "I'm excessively feeble. You go on, Bambi."
Another young deer limited by. "Bambi, run! Don't simply remain there in the event that you can run!" He took off like a breeze, and as Bambi ran along, he called behind him, "I will return for you, Gobo!" Bambi ran and ran. Before long, the sound that blasted as uproarious as thunder developed increasingly removed.

When Bambi came back to where Gobo had been, there was no hint of him, not, in any case, his tracks. Simply enormous tracks. Faline and her mom were walking about the spot. "What has happened to him?" howled Ena. Be that as it may, they all knew.

Weeks passed. Finally, little sprigs of new green grass sprung up through the day off. At that point, an ever-increasing number of tufts of green. What was left of the snow dissolved away? On Bambi's head, he could feel the heaviness of his fast-developing tusks.

As the trees and brambles turned green and the climate warmed, every one of the animals started to act so strangely. Winged creatures bounced around in pairs. Such huge numbers of animals enormous and little were two by two. His companion Skunk invested all his energy was with a young lady skunk and barely saw Bambi. Indeed, even his companion Hare appeared in a stupor, always staring at a young lady bunny and pounding his foot.

"What's befallen my companions?" said Bambi. "I am separated from everyone else." There was a stirring in the abandons him. There stood Faline. However, she was grown up now, as was he. Every one of them was thinking, "How extraordinary you look!" They looked at one another and grinned.

causeIt has been quite a while since we saw one another," said Faline.

"Truly, I know," said Bambi. They discussed bygone eras. "Do you played Tag on the glade?" said one. "Do you recollect every one of the berries on the shrubberies we ate?" said the other. The two appeared to see each other consummately.

A deer came up to them, and begin sniffing the air.

"Dear sister, don't you know me anymore?"

Faline and Bambi turned in awe. "Gobo!" They surged up to him in bliss.

"So no doubt about it!" said Bambi.

"Where have you been?" said Faline.

Gobo recounted his story. "I was with a Human. I have seen much more than all of, altogether." Dogs had discovered him when he lay in the day off, they woofed. The Human came and conveyed Gobo to where he lived. "Downpour may pour outside, however not inside where Humans live. It is constantly dry and warm! Furthermore, there is continually something to eat, as well – turnips, feed, potatoes, carrots – yum!"

"Weren't you apprehensive, however?" said Faline.

"No, the Human wouldn't hurt me. If he cherishes you, or in the event that you serve him, he's great to you," said Gobo. "They all adored me there. The children petted me."

The Great Old Buck walked out from the brambles. "What sort of band is that you have on your neck?"

"It's a bridle I wear," said Gobo. "It's an amazing privilege to wear the Human's strap."

"Be quiet!" said the Great Old Buck. "You poor thing." He turned and was gone.
One day when Gobo and Bambi were as one, they smelled the fragrance of a Human. "We should cover-up, without a moment's delay!" said Bambi. "No requirement for that," said Gobo. "Humans know me." Then at the same time, a sharp blast! Also, Gobo tumbled down.
Luckily, the Human never came after Gobo. Rather, when the aroma of the Human left, Bambi destroyed his companion to a verdant spot where he could laid and rest and be out of threat. Bambi comprehended what weeds his mom used to eat to recuperate an injury faster. As he carried the weeds to Gobo, he pondered, "For what reason should this consistently transpire?" Bambi stated, "Discover for yourself." Find out what?

Faline and Ena carried Gobo nourishment and chatted with him for a considerable length of time. Bambi regularly dropped by, as well, until Gobo was mended.
Seasons went back and forth. Bambi developed still taller. His prongs were almost fully developed at this point. At some point, Bambi found another admonition smell noticeable all around. It was a hot and smoky smell. A herd of crows surged overhead, cawing noisily. Fire!
Without a moment's delay, the animals were running, running, as fast as possible. It was difficult to flee from the fire. Sometimes it appeared to surge in from various bearings. Twilight passed by of blazes and smoke, and the fire started to slow down finally. The smell of fire was blurring, as well.
The Great Old Buck stepped before Bambi. His head was dark now, yet despite everything, he bore his prongs with satisfaction. "Accompany me," he said in a genuine way. "I need to give you something before I go."

He drove Bambi through the forested areas to a wore out the town. Blended alongside the smell of fire was the equivalent dreadful smell of Humans that had sent fear to their souls over and over.

"Try not to be alarmed," said the Old Buck. Consistently nearer, they went to the town. "See, Bambi," he said. There before them were many cabins. Every one was scorched, some nearly to the ground, others consumed for the most part on the rooftop. The town was unfilled.

"Bambi," said the Old Buck. "The places of the Humans get scorched by fire simply like the spots where we remain in the forested areas. The Human isn't above us. We are only the equivalent. Do you get me, Bambi?"

"Fire consumes the forested areas where we live, and it consumes the towns of Humans, as well," said Bambi. "We are not all that unique in relation to Humans."

"We both live under similar extraordinary power in this world," said the Great Old Buck.
"Indeed," said Bambi.
"Presently, I can go," said the Great Old Buck. "Try not to tail me. My time is up. Farewell, my child, I cherished you so."

Presently Bambi had become a full Buck himself. His tusks spiked and shined in the sun.

Sometimes he would visit the edge of the forested areas where he had spent his childhood. A portion of the path was still there. Once while meandering there, he saw Gobo and his sister, Faline. At the point when he saw Faline, his heart beat faster. He needed to hurry to her. He looked after her. At long last, she was no more. At that point, he heard the call of two little grovels.
"Mother! Mother!" they called.
"Wouldn't you be able to remain without anyone else's input?" said Bambi. The younger sibling and sister were a lot in the wonder of the incomparable Buck to reply. Bambi thought this little individual satisfies me. He helps me to remember the deer face I used to see when I glanced in the creek years prior. Maybe I'll meet him once more. The young lady is decent, as well. Faline resembled that once.

"Hear me out," said Bambi to the two grovels. "You should watch and tune in. Discover for yourself. You will be fine alone."

6. A Caterpillar's Voice

Once upon a time, a Caterpillar was out for a walk and went to a cavern. "My, my!" said Caterpillar. "This resembles a decent cavern!" Caterpillar glanced in the entryway of the cavern. "I don't see anybody in there," he said. "I will go in." Caterpillar headed inside.

Thus Caterpillar crept up over a stone. What's more, that was the place he nodded off. Directly at the extremely same time, Hare, who lived in that cavern, was likewise out for a walk. At the point when Hare got back home, she saw blemishes on the ground.

This woke up Caterpillar. Also, Caterpillar blasted in an extremely noisy voice, "It is I! Truly, I who stamps rhinos in the earth and steps elephants into dust!" Hare bounced about in dread.

"What can a little animal as me do with a beast who stamps rhinos and elephants?"

Before long, Jackal cruised by. Rabbit stated, "Companion Jackal, somebody has come inside my cavern! If there is no trouble, will you help me?" Jackal stated, "Indeed, I am glad to help." Jackal

went up to the cavern and yapped uproariously, "Who is in the place of my companion, Hare?" Caterpillar called out in a voice that shook the earth. "It is I! Truly, I who stamps rhinos in the earth, and steps elephants into dust!" On hearing this, Jackal thought in dread, "I can do nothing against such an animal!" And Jackal ran off as fast as possible.
At that point, Leopard cruised by. Rabbit told Leopard everything that had occurred. Panther stated, "I am greater than Jackal, and I am all the more uproarious." At the entryway of the cavern, Leopard hollered, "Who is in the place of my companion, Hare?" Caterpillar got back to similarly he had done previously. Panther was amazed. He thought, "If this animal stamps rhinos and elephants, I would prefer even not to consider what he could do to me!" And Leopard ran off fast.

Next, Rhino cruised by. "Everybody realizes how enormous and terrifying I am," snorted Rhino. He walked up to Hare's cavern. He grunted and pawed the ground with his enormous feet. Be that as it may, when Rhino asked who was inside the cavern and he heard Caterpillar's blasting answer, he stated, "This isn't great! He can stamp me into the earth? I am gone!"
"I am gone!" And Rhino fled, slamming through the forest."

Indeed, even Elephant attempted to help. In any case, similar to the others, when Elephant heard what Caterpillar needed to state, he realized he had no desire to be stepped underneath like residue. What's more, he ran off fast, as well.

Bunny didn't have the foggiest idea of what to do! At that point, Frog cruised by. "What's up?" said Frog, and Hare let him know. "Possibly, I can support you," said Frog. "I wish you could," said Hare. "In any case, Jackal attempted to help. What's more, Leopard attempted to help. Indeed, even Rhino and Elephant attempted to help. Furthermore, none of them could." "In any case," said Frog. "Allow me to attempt." T heard their names expressed, and they came up to observe what was happening. "What, you?" giggled Jackal. "You are excessively little!" "You can't help!" said Rhino. Every one of the animals snickered. "He needs to," said Hare.
"Why not let Frog attempt?"
Thus Frog went to the cavern entryway and asked who was inside. He got a similar answer as had been given to the others. At that point, Frog went all the closer and yelled, "I, who am the most grounded of all, have come finally. I am the person who stamps the individuals who stamp the rhinos! I am the person who steps underneath the individuals who step the elephants!"

At the point when Caterpillar inside Hare's cavernhey a heard this, he was afraid. He csee the shadow of Frog coming consistently nearer. He thought, "All things considered, I am just a caterpillar!" And Caterpillar crawled out of Hare's cavern, trusting that nobody would see him. In any case, they saw him!

"I could never fantasy about remaining in that cavern!" said Caterpillar with his nose noticeable all around. "A reverberation like that is dreadfully rough for an extravagant animal like me!" As Caterpillar sniffed away, the various animals chuckled at the difficulty such a little thing had given them.

7. The Mouse That Roared Story

Quite a long time ago in the jungle, there experienced an elderly person. He used to live in an old cabin. He was known for his mysterious forces, and he used to ponder throughout the day. At some point, the little mouse was meandering close to the jungle. He was eager. So he was searching for nourishment all over. He needed to eat something to fill his stomach.

All of a sudden, he saw that there was a fox pursuing him. He got scared. He needed to spare his life. Thus, he chose to go to the elderly person to request help. The poor mouse rushed towards the elderly person. At the point when he came to, he asked the elderly person, "Goodness, elderly person! It will be ideal if you help me! The fox is pursuing me. He will eat me!" The sort, elderly person, utilized his otherworldly powers and transformed the mouse into a tiger.

The tiger was not scared of anybody. He thundered uproariously and scared the fox away. The fox went dashing into the jungle. At that point, the tiger had a difference in heart. He turned into a pitiless animal. He used to inconvenience every one of the animals and execute them without being ravenous. It turned into his everyday employment to inconvenience every animal pointlessly.
He was dreadful that if the elderly person found that he was carrying out inappropriate things in the wake of turning into a tiger, at that point, the elderly person would transform him into a mouse by and by. Along these lines, he chose to proceed to murder the elderly person. The tiger went to the elderly person's hovel and saw that the elderly person was ruminating once more.

Before he could jump on him and murder him, the elderly person transformed him into a mouse by and by. The elderly person said to the mouse, "Mouse, you ought to be appreciative of me for sparing your life that day. Rather than being appreciative, you attempted to execute me!" Finally, the mouse understood his slip-up. Feeling embarrassed, he stated, "I am upset for not being appreciative enough to you for sparing my life. I didn't intend to do that!" To this, the elderly person stated, "Presently, you have the right to live like a mouse!"

8. Crocodile and Monkey Story

This is the Crocodile and Monkey Story. Some time ago, in a delightful jungle, there was an exquisite lake. In the lake, there carried on a huge yet delicate crocodile and on the close by tree carried on a brilliant monkey. The monkey and the crocodile were excellent companions.

Regular, the monkey would cull some succulent apples for the crocodile and offer them to him when he came to visit him toward the beginning of the day. Toward the evening, the crocodile would swim to the focal point of the lake and pick a few fishes and convey them back to the monkey. The two companions played together and talked for a considerable length of time.

At some point, the crocodile met the woman crocodile. At the point when the spouse of the crocodile heard that her better half had a monkey as a companion, she felt insatiable and needed to eat the monkey. That, prior night resting, woman crocodile requested the crocodile to get the core of the monkey with the goal that she would look increasingly lovely as she heard this someplace. She requested that he welcome the monkey in the lunch to their place where the woman crocodile would execute the monkey and eat his heart. The crocodile turned out to be miserable and calm. At long last, he made a guarantee to her better half that he would bring the monkey tomorrow.

The following day, when the monkey met the crocodile, he saw that something wasn't right. The crocodile approached him for a ride. The monkey immediately sat on the crocodile's back. The crocodile told the monkey that he guaranteed his significant other that he would bring the monkey as her lunch with the goal that she could turn out to be increasingly wonderful. The monkey was cunning to the point that he told the crocodile that he left his heart with the apples. The benevolent crocodile swam back to the tree. As the back came, the monkey bounced off the crocodile's back. The monkey said to him, "You were silly not exclusively to trust me yet additionally to what your significant other said!" Saying this, the monkey went into the jungle deserting the pitiful crocodile.

9. The Bowman And The Lion

A gifted bowman called the archer once chose to dive chasing deep in the forest. He was known for his precise point, and every one of the animals was very much aware of his abilities. aFrom the time they saw the bowman entering the forest, the animals started escaping the forest in search of places of refuge. They realized that if the bowman saw them, he could murder them with one shot of his bolt.

There was a lion in the forest. He didn't care for the manner in which every one of the animals started running for their lives. He chose to challenge the bowman. All things considered, he was the lord of the forest. He moved towards the course of the bowman. After observing the bowman, he thundered uproariously. The bowman was additionally outstandingly gifted in shooting bolts towards the bearing of sound.
He prepared his bow and bolt, and got out boisterously, "I send thee my flag-bearer. My delivery person ought to have the option to pass on you my capacities)". Saying this, the bowman shot a bolt toward the lion's thunder.

The bolt hit the lion and harmed him severely. Stunned by the unexpected assault, the lion lost his heart and started running for his life. A fox was observing every one of the occasions from a separation. It chose to have a word with the lion.

The fox halted the lion and disclosed to him that being the ruler of the jungle, it didn't teach him a thing or two to leave the battle like a defeatist. He ought to return and face the assailant with boldness.

The lion answered, "You counsel me futile, for in the event that he sends so dreadful an emissary, by what means will I tolerate the assault of the man himself? (While you encourage me to confront the bowman, simply delay and think for a minute. On the off chance that the delegate of the bowman was so deadly, simply envision how amazing and deadly would be his 'assault').
Moral: It is important to remain mindful of the individuals who can strike from a separation. Additionally, pick your consultants carefully.

10.THE LITTLE JACKALS AND THE LION

Once there was an incredibly huge jungle, and in the jungle, there was an extraordinary enormous Lion; and the Lion was lord of the jungle. At whatever point he needed anything to eat, all he needed to do was to come up out of his collapse the stones and earth and thunder. At the point when he had thundered a couple of times, all the little individuals of the jungle were startled to such an extent that they left their gaps and covering up places and ran, along these lines and that, to escape. At that point, obviously, the Lion could see where they were. Furthermore, he jumped on them, slaughtered them, and ate them up.

He did this so frequently that finally there was not a solitary thing left alive in the jungle other than the Lion, with the exception of two little Jackals,

- a little dad Jackal and a little mother, Jackal.

They had fled so often that they were very dainty and tired, and they couldn't run so fast anymore. Furthermore, one day the Lion was close to such an extent that the little mother Jackal developed alarmed; she stated, -
"Gracious, Father Jackal, Father Jackal! I believe our time has come! the Lion will, without a doubt, get us this time!"

"Pooh! garbage, mother!" said the little dad Jackal. "Come, we'll run on a piece!" And they ran, ran, ran exceptionally fast, and the Lion didn't get them that time.
In any case, finally, a day came when the Lion was closer still, and the little mother Jackal was startled going to death.

"Goodness, Father Jackal, Father Jackal!" she cried; "I'm certain our time has come! The Lion will eat us this time!"

"Presently, mother, don't you fuss," said the little dad Jackal; "you do similarly as I let you know, and it will be okay."
At that point what did those cleverness little Jackals do however grab hold of hands and run up towards the Lion, as though they had implied

To come constantly. At the point when he saw them coming, he stood up, and thundered in a horrible voice, -

"You hopeless little villains, come here and be eaten, on the double! For what reason did 't you precede?"
The dad Jackal bowed low.

"Undoubtedly, Father Lion," he stated, "we intended to precede; we knew we should precede, and we needed to precede; however every time we started to come, a shocking, extraordinary lion left the forested areas and thundered at us, and terrified us, so we fled."
"What do you mean?" thundered the Lion. "There's no other lion in this jungle, and you know it!"

"In fact, for sure, Father Lion," said the little Jackal, "I realize that is the thing that everyone thinks; except in fact and to be sure there is another lion! Also, he is as a lot greater than you as you are greater than I! His face is considerably more horrendous, and his thunder far, undeniably progressively frightful. Gracious, he is unquestionably more frightful than you!"

At that, the Lion stood up and thundered with the goal that the jungle shook.

"Take me to this lion," he said; "I'll gobble him up and afterward I'll gobble you up."

The little Jackals moved on ahead, and the Lion stalked behind. They drove him to a spot where there was around, profound well of clear water. They went around on one side of it, and the Lion stalked up to the next.

"He lives down there, Father Lion!" said the little Jackal. "He lives down there!"

The Lion approached and gazed down into the water, - and a lion's face glanced back at him out of the water!

At the point when he saw that, the Lion thundered and shook his mane and went on the defensive. Also, the lion in the water shook his mane and went on the defensive. The Lion shook his mane again and snarled once more, and made a horrible face. In any case, the lion in the water made similarly as awful a one, back. The Lion above could 't stand that. He jumped down into the well after the other lion.

Be that as it may, obviously, as you most likely arc aware well indeed, there was 't some other lion! It was just the appearance in the water!

So the poor old Lion fumbled about and flopped about, and as he could 't get up the lofty sides of the well, he was suffocated dead. What's more, when he was suffocated the little Jackals grabbed hold of hands and moved around the well, and sang, -

"The Lion is dead! The Lion is dead!

"We have murdered the incomparable Lion who might have executed us!

"The Lion is dead! The Lion is dead!

"Ao! Ao! Ao!"

11.THE COUNTRY MOUSE AND THE CITY MOUSE

When a little mouse who lived in the nation welcomed a little Mouse from the city to visit him, at the point when the little City Mouse plunked down to supper, he was astonished to find that the Country Mouse had nothing to eat aside from grain and grain.

"Truly," he stated, "you don't live well by any stretch of the imagination; you should perceive how I live! I have a wide range of fine things to eat each day. You should come to visit me and perceive that it is so decent to live in the city."
The little Country Mouse was happy to do this, and sooner or later, he went to the city to visit his companion.

The absolute in front of the pack that the City Mouse took the Country Mouse to see was the kitchen organizer of the house where he lived. There, on the most minimal rack, behind some stone containers, stood a major paper pack of dark-colored sugar. The little City Mouse chewed a gap clinched and welcomed his companion to snack for himself.

The two little mice snacked and snacked, and the Country Mouse thought he had never tasted anything so heavenly in his life. He was simply thinking how fortunate the City Mouse was when all of a sudden, the entryway opened with a blast, and in came the cook to get some flour.

"Run!" murmured the City Mouse.
Also, they ran as fast as they could to the little opening where they had come in. The little Country Mouse was shaking all over when they escaped securely, yet the little City Mouse stated, "That is nothing; she will come before long leave and afterward we can return."
After the cook had left and shut the entryway, they took delicately back, and this time the City Mouse had something new to appear: he took the little Country Mouse into a corner on the first-rate, where a major container of dried prunes stood open. After much pulling and pulling, they got an enormous dried prune out of the container on to the rack and started to snack at it. This was stunningly better than the dark-colored sugar. The little Country Mouse enjoyed the taste, so a lot of that he could scarcely snack sufficiently fast. At the same time, amidst their eating, there came a scratching at the entryway and a sharp, boisterous miaow!

"What is that?" said the Country Mouse. The City Mouse simply murmured, "Sh!" and ran as fast as he could to the gap. The Country Mouse pursued, you might make certain, as fast as possible. When they were out of risk, the City Mouse stated, "That was the old Cat; she is the best mouser around - on the off chance that she once gets you, you are lost."
"This is entirely horrible," said the little Country Mouse, "let us not return to the cabinet once more."

"No," said the City Mouse, "I will take you to the basement; there is something particular there."

So the City Mouse brought his little companion down the basement stairs and into a major cabinet where there were many racks. On the racks were containers of spread, and cheeses in sacks and out of packs. Overhead draped lots of hotdogs, and there were fiery apples in barrels remaining about. It smelled so wonderful that it went to the little Country Mouse's head. He ran along with the rack and snacked at a cheddar here, and a touch of margarine there, until he saw a particularly rich, delightful smelling bit of cheddar on a strange little sub a corner. He was simply on the purpose of placing his teeth into the cheddar when the City Mouse saw him.

"Stop! stop!" cried the City Mouse. "That is a snare!"

The little Country Mouse halted and stated, "What is a snare?"
"That thing is a snare," said the little City Mouse. "The moment you contact the cheddar with your teeth, something descends on your head hard, and you're dead."
The little Country Mouse took a gander at the snare, and he took a gander at the cheddar, and he took a gander at the little City Mouse. "In the event that you'll pardon me," he stated, "I figure I will return home. I'd preferably have grain and grain to eat and eat it in harmony and solace than have darker sugar and dried prunes and cheddar - and be alarmed to death constantly!"

So the little Country Mouse returned to his home, and there he remained an amazing remainder.

12.LITTLE JACK ROLL AROUND

Some time ago, there was a small young man who rested in a minor trundle-bed close to his mom's extraordinary bed. The trundle-bed
Had castors on it so it could be moved about, and there was nothing on the planet the young man preferred to such an extent as to have it rolled. At the point when his mom came to bed, he would cry, "Roll me around! Move me around!" And his mom would put out her hand from the huge bed and drive the little bed to and fro till she was drained. The young man would never get enough, so for this, he was called "Little Jack Roll around."
One night he had made his mom move him about till she nodded off, and that being said, he continued crying, "Roll me around! move me around!" His mom drove him about in her sleep until she fell too sufficiently slumbering; at that point, she halted. In any case, Little Jack Rollaround continued crying, "Roll around! Move around!"

Before long, the Moon peeped in at the window. He saw a clever sight: Little Jack Rollaround was lying in his trundle-bed, and he had set up one minimal fat leg for a pole and fastened the side of his small shirt to it for a sail, and saying, "Roll around! move around!" Slowly,
Gradually, the little trundle-bed vessel started to move; it cruised along the floor and up the divider and over the roof and down once more!

"More! More!" cried Little Jack Rollaround; and the little vessel cruised faster up the divider, over the roof, down the divider, and over the floor. The Moon snickered at sight; however, when Little Jack Rollaround saw the Moon, he got out, "Open the entryway, old Moon! I need to move through the town, with the goal that the individuals can see me!"

The Moon couldn't open the entryway, yet he shone in through the keyhole, in an expansive band. What's more, Little Jack Rollaround cruised his trundle-bed pontoon up the bar, through the keyhole, and into the road.
"Make a light, old Moon," he said; "I need the individuals to see me!"

So the great Moon made light and obliged him, and the little trundle-bed vessel went cruising down the avenues into the central avenue of the town. They moved past the town lobby and the school building and the congregation; however, no one saw little Jack Rollaround, on the grounds that everyone was in bed, asleep.

"For what reason don't the individuals come to see me?" he yelled.

High up on the congregation steeple, the Weather-vane replied, "It is no time for individuals to be in the boulevards; nice society are in their beds."

"At that point, I'll go to the forested areas, with the goal that the animals may see me," said Little Jack. "Tag along, old Moon, and make a light!"

The great Moon came and made a light, and they went to the forest. "Roll! Roll!" cried the young man, and the trundle-bed went trundling among the trees in the incredible wood, producing the chipmunks and startling the little leaves on the trees. The poor old Moon started to make some awful memories of it, for the tree-trunks impeded him so he couldn't go so fast as the bed, and each time he got behind, the young man called, "Hurry up, old Moon, I need the beasts to see me!"

Every one of the animals was asleep, and no one at all seen Little Jack Rollaround with the exception of an old White Owl, and all she said was, "Who are you?"
The young man didn't care for her, so he

Blew more enthusiastically, and the trundle-bed pontoon went cruising through the forest till it arrived at the apocalypse.

"I should return home now; it is late," said the Moon.

"I will go with you; make away!" said Little Jack Rollaround.

The thoughtful Moon caused a way to up to the sky, and up cruised the little bed into the middle of the sky. All the little brilliant Stars were there with their decent lights. What's more, when he saw them, that wicked Little Jack Rollaround started to prod. "Off the beaten path, there! I am coming!" he yelled and cruised the trundle-bed vessel directly at them. He knocks the little Stars both ways, everywhere throughout the sky, until all of them put his little light out and left it dull.

"Try not to treat the little Stars so," said the great Moon.

Be that as it may, Jack Rollaround just acted the more awful: "Get off the beaten path, old Moon!" he yelled, "I am coming!"

What's more, he controlled the little trundle-bed pontoon straight into the old Moon's face, and knock his nose!

This was a lot for the great Moon; he put out his large light, at the same time, and left the sky totally dark.

"Make a light, old Moon! Make a light!" yelled the young man. However, the Moon addressed never a word, and Jack Rollaround couldn't see where to guide. He went moving crosswise, here and there, everywhere throughout the sky, thumping into the planets and unearthing the mists, till he didn't have the foggiest idea where he was.

Abruptly he saw a major yellow light at the very edge of the sky. He thought it was the Moon. "Watch out, I am coming!" he cried and controlled for the light.

Be that as it may, it was not the caring old Moon by any means; it was the extraordinary mother Sun, simply coming up out of her home in the sea, to start her day's worth of effort.

"Aha, youngster, what are you doing in my sky?" she said. Furthermore, she picked Little Jack Rollaround up and tossed him, trundle-bed pontoon and all, into the center of the sea!

Also, I guess he is there yet, except if someone chose him once more.

13. The Last Dinosaurs

In a lost place that is known for tropical forests, over the main mountain in the area, caught inside an old volcanic cavity framework, experienced the last ever gathering of huge, fierce dinosaurs.

For a large number of years, they had endured every one of the progressions on Earth, and now, driven by the incomparable Ferocitaurus, they were intending to leave covering up and to rule the world again.

Ferocitaurus was a magnificent Tyrannosaurus Rex who had chosen they had invested an excessive amount of energy segregated from the remainder of the world. In this way, over a couple of years, the dinosaurs cooperated, crushing the dividers of the extraordinary hole. At the point when the work was done, every one of the dinosaurs carefully honed their hooks and teeth, in availability to threaten the world by and by.

At long last, from the highest point of certain mountains, they saw a community. Its homes and townsfolk appeared small specks. Never having seen individuals, the dinosaurs jumped down the mountainside, prepared to devastate whatever held them up...

Nonetheless, as they moved toward that little town, the houses were getting greater and greater... furthermore, when the dinosaurs, at last, showed up, it worked out that the houses were a lot greater than the dinosaurs themselves. A kid who was passing by stated: "Daddy! Daddy! I've discovered some minor dinosaurs! Would I be able to keep them?"

Furthermore, that is the way things are. The frightening Ferocitaurus and his companions wound up as pets for the town children. Perceiving how a large number of years of advancement had transformed their species into smaller person dinosaurs, they learned that nothing kept going forever and that you should consistently be prepared to adjust.

14. The Mocking Tiger

The tiger was sharp, speedy, and solid. He was continually ridiculing different animals, especially of the weak honey bee and the moderate and cumbersome elephant.
At some point, the animals were having a gathering in a cavern when there was an avalanche that sealed up the cavern entrance. Everybody anticipated that the tiger should spare them, yet he proved unable.
At last, the honey bee got away through a minor hole between the stones.
He took off in search of the elephant, who hadn't gone to the gathering since he was feeling tragic. The elephant came and moved the stones, liberating the animals.

The animals complemented both the elephant and the honey bee and were quick to be their companions. The last animal to leave the cavern was the tiger, shamefacedly. He learned his exercise, and from that very first moment, he just observed the positive qualities in the various animals.

15. Manute the Brave

"The best man in the entire clan is Manute the daring," everybody would state. You could see with your own eyes, whenever of the day, exactly how bold he was. He would hop to the ground from astonishing statures, and he would battle venomous snakes, he would get scorpions with his exposed hands, and could cut the palm of his own hand with a blade - without even a wince. They said the careful inverse about Potomac. Nobody had seen him get even a monkey.

At some point, they stumbled over one another in the forest, and Manute was indicating Pontoma, a coral snake he had quite recently gotten when there started a deluge, any semblance of which nobody had ever observed. The two of them raced to shield themselves under some thick foliage, and there they remained until the downpour had halted.
Be that as it may, when they were going to leave the asylum, they heard the thunder of a tiger, a ways off of just two or three meters. The foliage was thick and thick, and the tiger wouldn't have the option to overcome it to assault them. In any case, the tiger was nearly at the passage opening. In the event that it happened to come in and locate the two tribesmen there, they absolutely wouldn't get out alive. Manute was getting anxious. He needed to escape that tight gap, and stand up to the tiger in open space, where he could completely utilize his incredible chasing abilities. Potomac was motioning at him to keep still and be peaceful. However, Manute, tired of being left with a quitter, jumped out of the brush, astounding the tiger.
The tiger endured a few profound injuries, however before long recovered, and hurt Manute with two swipes of its paw, tossing him to the ground. The tiger stepped up, and jumped upon Manute, however Manute's lance, in the hands of Pontoma, intruded on the tiger's assault. The tiger dismissed, injured, yet the lance moved as fast as light emission, and with mind-blowing accuracy, harming the animal over and over, until it tumbled to the ground, dead.

Manute, stunned, and draining openly from his wounds, saw this while lying level on his back on the ground. At no other time had he seen anybody take on a tiger, and utilize the lance with such smoothness and quality, as he had seen Pontoma do a little while ago.

Neither of them said a thing. Manute's appreciative articulation required no words to be comprehended. Nor did they need words to think about Pontoma's injured hand or the way that they were leaving a tiger skin there in the forest.
From that day on, individuals steadily commented less on Manute's braveness. They thought possibly he was less valiant than previously. The most bizarre thing was that they presently saw that Manute's old lance was among Pontoma's things.

Be that as it may, Manute just grinned and recollected the day he learned that genuine courage lay not in searching out peril, however, in controlling one's dread when peril crosses your way.

16. The Mysterious Juggling Clown

Sometime in the distant past, a shuffling jokester went to a town. The comedian went from town to town, winning a minimal expenditure from his show. In that town, he started his demonstration in the square. While everybody was having fun, a devious kid started to ridicule the jokester, guiding him to leave the town. The yells and put-down made the comedian nervous, and he dropped one of his shuffling balls. Some others in the group started booing due to this mix-up, and at last, the jokester needed to leave rapidly.
He ran off, leaving four of the shuffling balls. In any case, neither the jokester nor his shuffling balls were in any capacity conventional. During that night, every single one of the balls mystically transformed into a devious kid, much the same as the person who had yelled the put-down — all with the exception of one ball, which transformed into another comedian. For the entire of the following day, the duplicates of the shrewd kid strolled around the town, raising hell for everybody. Toward the evening, the duplicate of the jokester started his shuffling appear, and something very similar occurred as the earlier day. In any case, this time, there were four shrewd young men yelling, rather than one. Once more, the jokester needed to run off, abandoning another four balls. Again, during the night, three of those balls transformed into duplicates of the mischievous kid, and one transformed into a comedian. Thus a similar story rehashed itself for a few days until the town was loaded up with underhanded young men who might leave nobody in harmony. The town older folks chose to put a conclusion to this. They ensured that none of the underhanded young men would lack respect or affront anybody. At the point when the jokester's show started, the older folks avoided the young men, in any event, making a squeak. So the jokester figured out how to complete his show, and could go through that night in the town.

That night, three of the duplicates of the underhanded kid vanished, and the equivalent occurred until just the comedian, and the first devious kid remained.

The kid, and everybody in the town, had been demonstrated exactly how far they could go. From that point on, rather than fleeing, that town bent over backward to ensure that guests would go through a decent day there. The locals had discovered exactly how much a modest voyaging comedian could educate with his show.

14. The Evil Goblins

Once upon a time, there was a posse of underhandedness goblins who lived in a forest. They invested a great deal of their energy ridiculing a poor elderly person who could now barely move, see, or hear. They demonstrated no regard for his age.

The circumstance turned out to be outrageous to the point that the Great Wizard chose to show the goblins a thing or two. He does magic, and from that minute, each affront they coordinated at the elderly person improved the elderly person, however, had the contrary impact on the troll who was doing the annoying. Obviously, the goblins thought nothing about what was occurring. The more they considered the man an "old moron," the younger and more keen of mind he became, while the troll who had yelled at him matured quickly, and turned into somewhat more absurd.

As time went on, those detestable goblins were getting awfully old, terrible, inept, and awkward... without acknowledging it. At long last, the Great Wizard enabled the goblins to see themselves, and, frightened, they saw that they had transformed into the nauseating animals we presently know as trolls.

They had been so bustling singling out the elderly person, that it had made them unequipped for seeing that their own demonstrations were transforming them into monsters. Also, when they at long last acknowledged what they had done, it was past the point of no return.

17. A Day With The Pigs

There was at one time a kid who might never get dressed when his folks instructed him to, nor would he put on what they needed him to after his shower. He wanted to dress in a lot more unusual way, yet most importantly, he got a kick out of the chance to take as much time as is needed. His folks were consistently in a surge and needed him to be much speedier. However, the kid didn't care for this, and he would back off considerably more.

At some point, his folks were in their standard rush, and they got so irate when he wouldn't dress, that they disclosed to him that he would need to go out exposed. The kid wouldn't fret this at all. So out they went.

While the kid was standing bare outside his home, trusting that his folks will bring the vehicle, along came the neighborhood pig rancher. The pig rancher was nearly deaf and had poor visual perception. That, yet he'd likewise neglected to put his glasses on that day. At the point when he saw the young man's pink skin, he thought it was one of his pigs. Also, with a touch of yelling, goading, and pushing, the rancher figured out how to recover the kid securely to a pigsty.

The kid fought the entire path there. However, as the rancher was practically hard of hearing, his grumblings didn't support him. Also, there he was for the entire day, living among the pigs, thought to be a pig, and sharing their nourishment and home.

At long last, however, his folks discovered him. The kid had such a lamentable day, that never again did he need to be confused with something besides a person. These days he's the first to get dressed and look consummately perfect and clean, much the same as those children in the garments lists.

18. A Ray of Moonlight

The forest wolf went through his evenings, yelling at the moon. He was ridiculing her, of how old she was, the means by which gradually she moved, and how minimal light she had. In a similar forest, when the yelling had halted, the little hedgehog would turn out to comfort the moon.
At some point, both the wolf and the hedgehog were a long way from home and were gotten unprepared by an incredible tempest. At the point when the tempest died down, the two animals were lost. As the moon turned out, the wolf started his typical crying, while the hedgehog was feeling dismal and scared at being lost.
In a little while, the hedgehog heard a voice calling him. However, he couldn't see anybody around. It was the moon, who was so thankful for the hedgehog's consistent assistance and counsel, that she needed to assist him with discovering his direction home. So the moon got together the entirety of her light into one single beam, to help tell the hedgehog the best way to get back securely.

The hedgehog showed up home in the early hours, while the wolf stayed lost, out in the haziness, and scared to death. At exactly that point, did he understand that all his impoliteness to the moon had been silly and barbarous? The moon didn't sparkle for him until the wolf requested absolution for his awful mentality, and vowed not to trouble anybody again like that.

19. Never Make Fun of a Rhino

Once, on the African fields, there carried on a grumpy rhino who was effectively irritated. At some point, a goliath turtle entered the rhino's domain ignorant. The rhino immediately went to the turtle, with the aim of disposing of it. The turtle was scared and pulled back into its shell.

At the point when the rhino requested that the turtle escape his domain, there was no detectable development. The rhino was extraordinarily irritated; he thought the turtle was tricking him. So he started slamming the shell to make the turtle turn out. No achievement and his blows got progressively savage. From a separation, it looked somewhat like a lone round of football, with the turtle as the ball.

A significant entertaining scene, it was, and a heap of monkeys before long assembled close by to appreciate it. They snickered relentless at the irate rhino and his battle with the turtle.

The rhino was enraged to the point that he didn't see that they were there. On he went until he needed to stop for one moment to get his breath.
Since he wasn't slamming the shell, he could hear the chuckling and kidding of the monkeys, who were ridiculing him all around you can envision.
Neither the rhino nor the turtle - who had shown up from his shell -, appreciated the way that a group of monkeys was taunting them.
In this way, they traded a knowing look, gestured, and the turtle returned inside his shell. This time the rhino discreetly withdrew a couple of steps, took a gander at the turtle, took a gander at the monkeys, took a run-up, and shot the monster turtle, with such a decent point, that it appeared as though he was utilizing the monkeys as skittles.

The 'strike' against the monkeys transformed that spot into something of a setback ward for mandrills. There they all lay, covered in cuts and wounds, and not by any means a grin crossed their lips. In the meantime, off went the rhino and the turtle, grinning like old companions... and keeping in mind that the monkeys were putting on their staying mortars, their boss acknowledged it was about time they found a superior method to entertain themselves than ridiculing others.

20. The Frog King Fairy Tale Story

In times past, when wishing still helped one, there carried on a ruler whose little girls were all delightful. However, the youngest was lovely to such an extent that the sun itself, which has seen so a lot, was astounded at whatever point it shone in her face. Nearer to the ruler's stronghold lay an extraordinary dim forest, and when the day was exceptionally warm, the lord's child went out into the forest and plunked somewhere around the side of the cool wellspring, and when she was exhausted she took a brilliant ball, and hurled it on high and got it, and this ball was her preferred toy.

Presently it so happened that on one event, the princess's brilliant ball didn't fall into the little hand which she was holding available, yet on to the ground past, and folded straight into the water. The ruler's little girl tailed it with her eyes. However, it evaporated, and the very much was profound, so profound that the base couldn't be seen. At this, she started to cry and cried stronger and stronger, and couldn't be consoled. Also, as she along these lines deplored somebody said to her, "What distresses you, lord's little girl? You sob so that even a stone would show feel sorry for."

She looked round to see the other side from whence the voice came, and saw a frog extending forward its large, terrible head from the water. "Ok, old water-splasher, is it you," she stated, "I am sobbing for my brilliant ball, which has fallen into the well." "Be tranquil, and don't sob," addressed the frog, "I can support you, yet what will you give me on the off chance that I bring your toy up once more?" "My garments, my pearls and gems, and even the brilliant crown which I am wearing." The frog replied, "I couldn't care less for your garments, your pearls, and gems, nor for your brilliant crown, however in the event that you will cherish me and let me be your partner and play-individual, and sit by you at your little table, and eat off your brilliant little plate, and drink out of your little cup, and sleep in your little bed - on the off chance that you will guarantee me this I will go down underneath, and present to you your brilliant ball up once more."

"Goodness, yes," said she, "I guarantee all of you wish, on the off chance that you will, however, present to me my ball back once more." But she thought, "How the senseless frog talks. Everything he does is to sit in the water with different frogs and croak. He can be no ally to any individual."

The frog when he had gotten this guarantee, put his head into the water and sank down, and in a brief time came swimming up again with the ball in his mouth, and tossed it on the grass. The lord's girl was enchanted to see her pretty toy again, and got it, and fled with it. "Pause, pause," said the frog. "Take me with you. I can't run as you can." But what did it profit him to shout his croak, croak, after her, as noisily as possible? She didn't hear it out, yet ran home and before long overlooked the poor frog, who had to return into his well once more.

The following day when she had seated herself at table with the lord and every one of the retainers and was eating from her brilliant little plate, something came crawling splish sprinkle, splish sprinkle, up the marble staircase, and when it had got to the top, it thumped at the entryway and cried, "Princess, youngest princess, open the entryway for me." She raced to see who was outside; however, when she opened the entryway, there sat the frog before it. At that point, she hammered the entryway to, in an incredible flurry, plunked down to supper once more, and was very alarmed. The ruler saw obviously that her heart was thumping viciously, and stated, "My child, what are you so scared of? Is there perchance a mammoth outside who needs to divert you?" "Ah, no," answered she. "It is no monster; however, an appalling frog."

"What does a frog need with you?" "Ah, dear dad, yesterday as I was in the forest sitting by the well, playing, my brilliant ball fell into the water. Also, on the grounds that I cried in this way, the frog brought it out again for me, and in light of the fact that he so demanded, I guaranteed him he ought to be my buddy. However, I never figured he would have the option to leave his water. Also, presently he is outside there, and needs to come into me."
Meanwhile, it thumped a subsequent time, and cried, "Princess, youngest princess, open the entryway for me, do you not realize what you said to me yesterday by the cool waters of the well. Princess, the youngest princess, open the entryway for me."

At that point said the ruler, "That which you have guaranteed must you perform. Proceed to give him access." She proceeded to open the entryway, and the frog bounced in and pursued her, bit by bit, to her seat. He sat and cried, "Lift me up next to you." She deferred until finally, the Lord told her to do it. When the frog was on the seat, he needed to be on the table, and when he was on the table, he stated, "Presently, push your brilliant little plate closer to me that we may eat together." She did this. However, it was anything but difficult to see that she didn't do it energetically. The frog delighted in what he ate, yet pretty much every significant piece she took stifled her. Finally, he stated, "I have eaten and am fulfilled, presently I am drained, convey me into your little room and prepare your little luxurious bed, and we will both rests and rest."

The ruler's girl started to cry, for she feared the virus frog, which she didn't prefer to contact, and which was present to sleep in her truly, clean little bed. Be that as it may, the lord became irate and stated, "He who helped you when you were in a difficult situation should not a while later to be loathed by you." So she grabbed hold of the frog with two fingers, conveyed him upstairs, and put him in a corner, however, when she was in bed he crawled to her and stated, "I am drained, I need to sleep just as you, lift me up or I will tell your dad." At this, she was horribly furious, and took him up and tossed him energetically against the divider. "Presently, will you hush up, accursed frog," said she. In any case, when he tumbled down, he was no frog yet a lord's child with kind and wonderful eyes. He by her dad's will was currently her dear buddy and spouse. At that point, he disclosed to her how he had been beguiled by a devilish witch and how nobody could have conveyed him from the well, however, herself, and that to-morrow they would go together into his realm.

At that point, they rested, and next morning when the sun got up them, a carriage came driving up with eight white steeds, which had white ostrich quills on their heads, and were bridled with brilliant chains, and behind stood the young ruler's hireling Faithful Henry. Steadfast Henry had been so despondent when his lord was changed into a frog, that he had made three iron groups be laid round his heart, in case it should overflow with distress and misery. The carriage was to lead the young lord into his realm. Loyal Henry helped them both in, and set himself behind once more, and was loaded with bliss in view of this liberation. What's more, when they had driven an almost the lord's child heard a breaking behind him as though something had broken. Again and by and by while they were en route, something split, and each time the ruler's child thought the carriage was breaking. However, it was just the groups that were springing from the core of Faithful Henry since his lord was liberated and was cheerful.

Santa Claus Does Not Forget

Bertie was a generally excellent kid. He was benevolent, obedient, honest, and unselfish. He had, in any case, one incredible shortcoming— he generally overlooked.

Regardless of how important the task, his answer consistently was, "I overlooked." When he was sent with a note to the dress-creator, his mom would discover the note in his pocket around evening time. On the off chance that he was sent to the store in an extraordinary rush, to get something for tea, he would return late without the article, however, with his typical answer.

His dad and mom talked about the issue over and concluded that something must be done to cause the young man to recall.

Christmas was close, and Bertie was occupied with making out a rundown of things that Santa Claus was to bring him.

"Santa Claus may overlook a portion of those things," said his mom.

"He can't," answered Bertie; "for I will compose sled, and skates, and drum, and violin, and every one of the things on this paper. At that point, when Santa Claus goes to my stocking, he will discover the rundown. He can see it and put the things in as fast as he peruses."

Christmas morning came, and Bertie was up at sunrise to perceive what was in his legging. His mom avoided him as long as she could, for she realized what Santa Claus had done.

At last, she heard him accompanying moderate strides to her room. Gradually he opened the entryway and came towards her. He grasped a rundown, especially longer than the one he had made out. He put it in his mom's hand, while tears of disillusionment tumbled from his eyes.

"See what Santa Claus left for me, yet I figure he may have given me one thing other than."

His mom opened the roll. It was a rundown of the considerable number of tasks Bertie had been approached to accomplish for a half year. Toward the finish of all was composed, in staring capitals, "I FORGOT."

Bertie sobbed for 60 minutes. At that point, his mom revealed to him they were all going to grandpas. Just because he would see a Christmas-tree, maybe something may be developing there for him.

It was unusual to Bertie, yet on grandpa's tree, he discovered all that he had composed on his rundown. Is it accurate to say that he was relieved of his negative behavior pattern? Not at the same time, yet when his mom saw that he was especially lax, she would state, "Recall, Santa Claus remembers."

21. A Wish For Christmas

Prior tonight, Christmas music folded over Matthew like an enchantment cover. Children and grown-ups of every kind imaginable rushed and yelled all through the shopping center.
It was energizing to see Christmas trees wearing all hues, hockey hardware, and trains. Computer games and toy troopers dissipated like snowflakes crosswise over presentation tables.
"Quit crying, I can't bear the cost of that!" one grown-up said. In the parking garage, Matthew couldn't close out irate voices. "Hello, you! That is my spot!"

Presently it was Christmas Eve, and Matthew remained by his bedroom window. From his second-floor window, Victoria Park looked tranquil.

"This ought to be a cheerful time," Matthew stated, tapping his feline, Boots. Victoria Park was in the focal point of the town, loaded up with climbing trails.

Mother gave him a colossal grin as she hung over and kissed him goodnight. "What unique present would you like for Christmas, Matthew?" she inquired.

"Tranquility on earth," he murmured.
"Where did you get such a genuine idea?" she inquired.
His answer was a monster embrace. He realized wishes should be a mystery. However, his mother was extraordinary.

Sleepy eyes shut as the clock ticked towards 12: 00 PM. By 11:00 PM, Matthew heard a sound first floor. Being an inquisitive kid, he got up and went to explore.
It seemed like a pooch, crying outside the front entryway. Is it true that it was a ravenous stray? Subsequent to getting a plate of leftover dinner from the ice chest, he opened the entryway. Matthew nearly fell in reverse as he saw a dim wolf. Its gigantic mouth was unguarded with a kind of glad gasping.

Oddly enough, Matthew wasn't apprehensive.

Kid and animal stared at one another. Matthew understand in his heart he was to head off to someplace with this animal. He discreetly returned upstairs, put on boots, and comfortable garments. Remember gloves and a cap.

When he returned, three additional wolves held up outside. What's more, this young kid, encompassed by four wolves, headed down the road.

A neighbor looked out her window, and let out an uproarious GASP. Subsequent to getting her telephone call, the Truro Police Department sent an earnest message: "Kid grabbed by wolves!"

A Cab driver shouted into his CB radio, "Wolves in the city!" Late-night walkers hurried to their homes and bolted the entryways. Noisy yelling started between neighbors here and there Park and Rosewyn Streets.

The wolf head went across the road and entered Victoria Park, with its 1,000 sections of land of woods. Matthew pursued. He realized this way prompted the little lake.

At this point, a group had assembled on the walkway. "That way!" somebody yelled, highlighting the Park Entrance. Officials from two Police vehicles left at that point joined everybody heading for the recreation center.

Christmas eve festivities were cleared from their psyches like residue balls. Sparing a young man from wild animals was substantially more important.

Not a long way ahead, four wolves held up as Matthew leaned against a birch tree. Inside his heart, Matthew realized he was on a unique strategy. The wolves appeared to know precisely where they were going.

They started to run when they heard the tramp of numerous feet. Yelling words were a piece of a developing horde of individuals. Some conveyed thick branches, and others had play clubs.

Dread was in their souls.

Maybe the entire town was progressing. They deserted extravagant Christmas treats and pretty designs. In any event, preparing for Santa was overlooked. What was more important now than protecting a young man on Christmas Eve?

Matthew saw an enormous number of animals on the path. Quills from crows, chick-a-dees, and ducks vacillated all over.

"Animals in the forest are generally nervous around individuals," father once said.

All of a sudden, the wolf chief halted then raised his nose. A penetrating "OWWWOOUUU" was his sign for different wolves to participate.

Matthew could see the forest topping off with more animals and winged creatures. Bigger trees resembled a clothesline for canaries, partridges, and owls.

Each animal and flying creature he knew from his school library appeared to be here. Behind bushes and trees were coyotes, hares and beaver, even mice and deer. Bear and moose were additionally here.

A multitude of individuals from the town was astounded to see such a significant number of untamed life sights. "OOHS" and "AAHS" originated from individuals, all things considered, shapes, and sizes. There were such a large number of animals and feathered creatures to check.

As though on a sign, every grown-up put sticks and polished ash on the ground. This exceptional quiet in the forest was something they would not like to fail.

What's more, they tuned in as four wolves wailed welcome to the night sky. The moon shone its electric lamp bar upon Matthew and the wolves. Everybody could see the kid was fine. Also, he wasn't apprehensive adjacent to four shaggy wolves.

Softly, a murmuring emerged from a great many trees.

Fluttering wings lifted gradually, at that point quickly, causing echoes of 'Whooshing' all through the forested areas.

Each appendage shuddered.
Winged creatures and animals participate with their own calls, making a melodic orchestra. Nut case tunes lifted gloriously into the sky. Deer included 'blowing' sounds intended to calm their young.

What's more, many beaver slapped ripped tails as they dove like bolts into the supply of water.

Men, ladies, and children wheezed in wonder as a blend of captivating sounds caught their ears. Music was about affection for the forest, to live in harmony, one with another.

It was a message felt by every human, occupying void spaces in their souls. Everything was quiet as fog floating through the trees.

At that point quietly as though a twirly doo had been raised, all animals and flying creatures were still. Their singing, venturing far into the sky and past the slopes, finished.

Tolerant grown-ups could scarcely hold in their energy.

As though that equivalent inconspicuous mallet whirled, a multitude of children's voices started to sing. They gladly stood and sent their own message of harmony. It emerged from the forest as a brilliant wave.

Grown-ups participate, wishing to be a piece of this incredible ensemble. As though by enchantment, animals and flying creatures likewise met up in agreement.

The forest shook with amazing sounds, abnormal in their conveyance, however ascending as a stairway to the stars. Animals of hiding and plumes, alongside people, conveyed a message of affection and tranquility on earth.

It was currently Christmas morning!

22. A Perfect Christmas

Claudio was extremely content with the manner in which the work had been apportioned. Of everything that required getting ready for the introduction of Jesus, he had been given 'the speaker.' In any case, it wasn't only any speaker: it was the speaker through which the voices of the holy messengers and God himself would be heard on Earth from Heaven.

Claudio was only a standard blessed messenger yet had been fortunate on the grounds that the main part of the important errands had been given to the most noteworthy and splendid lead celestial hosts and to other increasingly senior heavenly attendants. As everybody definitely knew, he was something other than a beguiling holy messenger: he was additionally a genius with innovation, which is the reason they figured he would be perfect for making such an entangled gadget.

Claudio had a thousand thoughts for the plan in his mind, and he set to work right away. He wasn't working sometime before Raphael, one of his preferred chief heavenly messengers, went along.

"Would you be able to please give us a hand with the royal residence, Claudio? We need an entryway that opens naturally for Mary and Joseph."

"Obviously!" – He stated, energetically as ever – "this can pause."
It took Claudio a few days to complete the confounded entryway, and much more to finish different occupations that Raphael continued requesting that he do.They manufactured a castle deserving of the best ruler on Earth. It was great to such an extent that, when nobody was looking, the holy messengers left paradise to appreciate it.
Claudio was strolling back so he could take a shot at his speaker when Michael, the chief heavenly messenger, spotted him from a far distance.
"Claudio, would you be able to please assist us with the completing contacts in the closet? At the point when the ensemble sings, we need the garments of those tuning in to sparkle with gold, valuable stones, and vivid lights and the garments of Mary, Joseph, and the Son of God to influence with the musicality of the music."
"What a phenomenal thought, Miguel! That will be stunning. I'll be there immediately."
Because it took a few days to complete the outfits, they couldn't have made much else lovely. Blessed messengers originated from each side of the universe to wonder about their magnificence and salute Michael energetically.
Gabriel likewise asked Claudio to assist him with the lights and audio effects for the great ensemble. At that point, the seraphs showed up requesting bunches of help, as did enormous quantities of senior heavenly attendants with employments so important that Claudio had no real option except to help them. Everything was great. The heavenly attendants were upbeat and complimented each other gladly. That equivalent night, the eve of the introduction of the baby Jesus, they celebrated with a major gathering.

In any case, Claudio couldn't go. After so much work, he recollected that he had his very own business to do - the speaker-which he had still not started! Alone and in a rush, Claudio took a shot at his speaker and could hear the ambient melodies from the gathering.

"Hi, my dear Claudio. What are you doing here and not at the gathering?"

The little heavenly attendant felt embarrassed and, keeping down the tears, demonstrated him the incompletely completed speaker.

"I see. I realize that you were caught up with helping other people. Be that as it may, is nobody coming to support you?"

"All things considered, they are celebrating at the large party, and they merit it," addressed Claudio. "They have buckled down, and everything has turned out splendidly. Likewise, they couldn't assist me with a night in the event that they needed to: this speaker is entangled."

"Gee" was the main thing God said as he pivoted. He didn't appear to be upbeat.

Claudio was alarmed. He realized that the main way he would arrive in time as if God has chosen to support him; however, he was too humiliated even to consider asking. As though he had guessed what he might be thinking, God went to Claudio and stated:

"Indeed, do as well as can be expected, however, ensure it is extremely noisy."

Claudio didn't have time. He had quite recently wrapped up the pieces together in time, and he figured out how to arrive at his place just barely, similarly as Gabriel was giving the sign to start. The ensemble cleared their voices, and for a subsequent everybody was taking a gander at Claudio. He shut his eyes, said a supplication, and put the speaker on full volume.

BOOOOOOM!!!

An immense blast shook Heaven as it opened up to send the blessed messengers' psalm to Earth. The blast was extraordinary to such an extent that it resembled a seismic tremor or a sea tempest on Earth, devastating every one of the arrangements. The royal residence crumbled totally aside from the remaining parts of a couple of dividers. The spot felt chilly, awkward, grimy, and messy. Indeed, even the delightful garments of all who were there to observe the birth flew over the air, presently just clothes. In merely seconds, all that stayed flawless were the voices of the grand ensemble and a brilliant blaze from the gigantic speaker, which was gradually consuming.

Nobody in Heaven challenged state anything. Claudio was exceptionally humiliated. Everybody was seeing him in pity and dissatisfaction, yet they also were humiliated for having disregarded him all. Simply then, Jesus was conceived yet rather than the calls of a baby, which was what everybody was expecting, glad giggling filled Heaven and Earth. It was infectious giggling, telling them that, despite the fact that things had turned out inadequately, God was content with the arrangements done generally by Claudio, who had overlooked his very own issues to help every other person.

What's more, as though they had expected something like this would occur, the three chief heavenly messengers murmured to themselves: "This is genuinely God's way: everything has turned out great."

The Little Christmas Star

Of the considerable number of stars that sparkle in the sky, there had consistently been one that was more brilliant and more wonderful than the others. The entire sky's planets and stars glanced on in appreciation, considering what could be the important strategic this star was to complete. What's more, the star itself did the very same, mindful of its own exceptional magnificence.
The theory finished when a gathering of blessed messengers went to the star:

- "Rush. Your time has shown up, and the Lord gets upon you to do an important strategic."
What's more, the star went as fast as he could and discovered that her crucial to show where the most important occasion in history would occur.
The star was loaded up proudly and dressed in her most wonderful ensemble of flicker and bedazzlement. She continued to pursue the blessed messengers, who might show her the opportune spot. The star shone with such quality and magnificence that she was seen from all pieces of the World, thus much so a gathering of shrewd men chose to pursue her, realizing that she should point something important.

For a considerable length of time, the star pursued the blessed messengers, demonstrating the way, and she was anxious to discover what place she would enlighten. Be that as it may, when the heavenly attendants halted, and with incredible happiness said, "Here it is!" the star could barely handle it. There were no royal residences, no strongholds or manors, no gold or gems. Just a little, half-surrendered, filthy, foul stable.

- "Gracious, no! Not that! I can not squander my sparkle and excellence, illuminating a spot this way! I was conceived for an option that is more prominent than this!"
What's more, however, the holy messengers attempted to quiet her, the star's wrath developed and developed. Thus much pride and self-importance rose inside her that she started to consume. What's more, in this manner, she expended herself and vanished.
Indeed, what an issue! There were just a couple of days left before the pivotal turning point, and they were without a star. The holy messengers, in a frenzy, hurried to Heaven to mention to God what had occurred. In the wake of intuition for a minute, God stated:
- "all things considered, search for the littlest, generally modest and cheerful of the considerable number of stars you can discover, and bring it here."
Amazed by request, however unquestioning, in light of the fact that the Lord frequently did this sort of thing, the holy messengers flew through the sky in search of the littlest, most upbeat star. It was a minor star, as little as a grain of sand. He understood so little that he gave no significance to his splendor, and he invested his entire energy chuckling and talking with his companions, the greatest stars. At the point when this star was brought to the Lord, he was told:

- "The absolute best star in creation, the most superb, the most splendid has flopped because of its pride. I imagined that you, the most modest and cheerful of the considerable number of stars, ought to be the one picked to have its spot and illuminate the most important occasion ever: the introduction of baby Jesus in Bethlehem."

The star was loaded up with so much feeling and happiness that he had just landed over Bethlehem, drove by the heavenly attendants, before he understood that his splendor was unimportant and that, anyway much he attempted, he couldn't enlighten things far superior to a firefly could.
- "Alright,"
He said to himself.
- "Why I didn't think before tolerating this task? I'm the littlest star there is! It is absolutely incomprehensible for me to do just as that incredible sparkling star ... Its disgrace! I'm going to destroy an open door that every one of the stars in the sky would have wanted to have had ..."

At that point, he reconsidered, "every one of the stars in the sky." obviously, they couldn't want anything more than to partake in something like this! Also, decisively, the start took to the skies with a message for every one of his companions:

- "On December 25th, at 12 PM, I need to impart to all of you the best wonder that can exist for a star: to illuminate the introduction of God! I will anticipate you in the little town of Bethlehem, by a little steady."

Also, for sure, none of the stars dismissed this liberal greeting. Such a large number of stars combined, that they framed the most excellent Star of Christmas that could ever be seen, despite the fact that the little star couldn't be seen in the midst of all the brightness. What's more, cheerful at his phenomenal assistance, and as a prize for his quietude and liberality, God changed this little courier into a wonderful falling star, and gave him the endowment of conceding wishes each time saw his excellent path sparkling in the night sky was seen.

OTHER BEDTIME STORIES

1. A Seaside Adventure (Ears Mouse)

Some time ago, It was an excellent sunny day, and Ears Mouse was eating a flawless thick cut of handcrafted toast, with his extremely most loved natively constructed Danny Jim. He had made the Danny Jim himself from organic products that had fallen the past pre-winter, and it had turned out exceptionally decent. He had the top area of his front entryway all the way open, and the Sun was sparkling straight into his kitchen. He could feel the glow of the Sun all over and contemplated internally, "this will be a blistering day." He could hear a great deal of movement outside his home as the numerous creatures in Oak View woods went here, and there the path is scavenging for nourishment.

Tap, he heard on the base of his entryway. He, at that point, heard some light scratching, and afterward, a dark round thing flew over the top – Ears Mouse knew straight away that it was Harry Hedgehog's nose as this was something he did a ton.

"Morning, Harry," Ears Mouse said.

"Morning Ears Mouse," Harry stated, "it's such an excellent day, and would it say it isn't"?

"Truly, in reality, it is," said Ears Mouse.

"I have recently been to see our different companions in the woodland and have inquired as to whether they extravagant a day at the seashore," Harry said "it's likely the last decent day that we will have this Summer – so best to take advantage of it" he proceeded. "are you available?" Harry asked Ears, Mouse.

Ears mouse could consider loads of errands that he expected to do around the house, as he expected to fix a couple of things before the Autumn and Winter showed up, anyway he took a gander at Harry who had a major smile all over thinking about the enjoyment they would all have at the Seaside. Ears Mouse couldn't frustrate Harry and the others, and inside he truly needed to go himself. "Presently, that sounds an awesome thought," said Ears Mouse " is every other person available"?

Harry didn't have to respond to that question, as simply then, the entirety of his different companions showed up at his front entryway. Olivia Owl was currently roosted over the entryway. They had all been tuning in to Harry and Ears Mouse trusting that Ears Mouse would state yes – as it would not be the equivalent without Ears Mouse. It generally appeared to be a superior adventure when he was there.

The entirety of different creatures, aside from Olivia, had sunglasses on and held basins and spades, and each had a backpack with beverages and nourishment.

"We believed that we should go to Shell Island seashore," said Molly, "it is by a wide margin the most delightful seashore". "isn't that a piece too far to even think about walking," said Ears Mouse, "particularly on such a hot day like today and with every one of these basins, spades, and backpacks to convey"?

"Ohhh – I guess you are correct, Ears Mouse," answered Molly, looking disillusioned.

"I have a thought," said Hammy Hamster, "we could inquire as to whether he might want to come also. I know where we can get a few carrots for him to eat to give him vitality for the voyage."

Everyone imagined that it would be an extraordinary thought. They all realize that Alex could be somewhat difficult and cranky some of the time, despite the fact that they were all acceptable companions with him, and he generally is by all accounts feeling better on the off chance that he could eat a few carrots first.

When Ears Mouse had pressed his backpack and put on his straw cap and sunglasses, they all set off with Hammy Hamster driving the best approach to where the carrots were put away. The carrots were in an old wooden, it was shed at the edge of a field, and there was a little opening toward the side of the shed – sufficiently huge for Hammy to slither in. He passed out a couple of carrots to the others, and Molly and Sid put them into their backpack as they were bigger than different creatures.

Sitting in the following field was Alex Donkey. They all drew nearer Alex and mentioned to him what an extraordinary spot Shell Island seashore would be and that they would have some good times. "Are there any carrots there?" asked Alex Donkey. "Goodness YES," said Sid Squirrel rapidly before any of the others could answer, "there are some under the shells on the seashore" . Sid realized he ought not to lie. However, he additionally realized that on the off chance that Alex realized that they had carrots in their backpacks, at that point, he would request them once in a while not want to do anything a while later.

"Yum – carrots," said Alex, "alright – I'm in," said Alex. "Horray" the others yelled – bouncing into the air – Freddy Frog dealing with the biggest hop. Alex set down in the grass, advised everybody to climb onto his back, and afterward, he found a workable pace. At the point when he found a good pace, Sid Squirrel bounced onto it, opened it to let Alex out onto the track, and afterward shut it. He, at that point, bounced onto Alex's back once more.

Olivia Owl, drifting above, said that she would direct them all to the seashore as it was quite a while since they were last there. While it was distinctly about a mile or so, it would have taken a large portion of them the entire day to arrive and one more day to get back if Alex had not tagged along. With Alex doing the entirety of the strolling, it was just a brief time before they could see the stunning blue ocean and the brilliant sand in see.

At the point when they landed at the seashore, Alex strolled around a piece until they had picked a pleasant spot close to a sand ridge. Alex plunked down on his base, and the creatures all slid down his back like a slide in a carnival. "Wheeeeee," they all said as they slid down into the sand.

Molly Mole and Harry Hedgehog began to spread out an outing cover while their different companions ran, bounced and flew down to the coastline. Ears Mouse plunged his toes into the ocean similarly as a wave went out – "Ouuuuuu," that is somewhat cool, he said. Freddy Frog said that he didn't care for salty ocean water as it made him tingle. Alex strolled gradually along the shore to chill himself off, and afterward, he sat in the water. Simply then, an enormous wave came in, and he was not quick enough to find a good pace thumped over. He immediately found a good pace, and anybody had ever observed Alex move in constantly that they had known him. He, at that point, ran onto the dry sand. Different creatures giggled for some time, yet when Alex chose to get himself dry by shaking himself, they all got shrouded in ocean water and sand.

Ears Mouse nearly got captured by a wave; however, fortunately, Olivia Owl swooped down in time and lifted him out of the water and onto the dry seashore. "Much obliged to you," said Ears Mouse to Olivia, "no issue," said Olivia.

"Anyone hungry, " Molly Mole yelled. She had put the entirety of the beautiful nourishment and beverages on the cover. There was bread, cheeses, worms, creepy crawlies, grain, milk, and water. Ears Mouse had likewise brought a portion of his home-made cake and scones.

Alex Donkey, at that point, recollected the guarantee of carrots. "Sid," said Alex, "where did you say the carrots would be"? At the point when no one was looking, Sid had placed a few carrots in the sand and had put enormous shells over them. "They live under shells," said Sid, "examine check whether you can discover them."

Alex lifted a couple of shells with his foot and immediately discovered a few carrots. He moved a couple of additional with his nose and discovered some more. He was flabbergasted that carrots developed under shells as he had never known about that. The others snickered at this so much it hurt.

When they had all completed lunch, they chose to play a few games on the seashore. Molly had brought an old tennis ball she had discovered covered in the ground when she had been burrowing under the ground. They tossed this to one another until Harry Hedgehog missed it, and it arrived on the spines on his back and burst.

"We should play another game," said Freddy Frog, "how about we see who can bounce the most noteworthy." "Nooo," they all stated, "you generally win that one," said Harry.

"I know," said Molly, "we should see who can locate the most intriguing thing on the seashore". "Extraordinary thought," said Sid Squirrel, and they all concurred.

Alex, however, that carrots would be an intriguing find; thus, he began to look under each shell that he could see on the seashore. Ears Mouse found a decent shell which, when he held it to his ear, he could hear the sound of waves – or would it say it was genuine waves he was hearing?

Harry found a decent bit of kelp with huge round darker air pockets, which popped on the off chance that he sat on it. Molly found an exquisite round and smooth stone, which she figured she would carry home to help her to remember the seashore. Olivia found a decent quill from a seagull which she would bring home for her home.

Sid Squirrel had meandered down the seashore a piece and afterward climbed a sand rise. As he came over the top, he couldn't accept his eyes. There before him was a monster shell with a top and a base. He had never observed a shell so huge. It was large to such an extent that he imagined that he might have the option to fit into it.

Inevitably the entirety of the creatures came back to the outing territory to perceive what each other had found; anyway, there was no indication of Sid. They all concluded that they better search for him, and Alex Donkey set down to let them jump on his back. Alex strolled here and there the seashore and afterward began to climb the sand rises. "Stop," said Ears Mouse, "I can hear a clamor like Sid yelling" – Ears Mouse generally had excellent hearing because of his huge ears. "Over toward that path," he stated, pointing toward one of the sandhills.

Alex climbed the sand ridge with the others clinging to his hide, so they didn't tumble off. At the point when he found a workable pace of the ridge, they all observed the huge shell. "Amazing," said Harry, "I've never observed a shell that size," and the others concurred. They could see that the shell had a top and a base; however, it was shut.

"Are you in there?" said Ears Mouse, thumping on the shell. "Indeed," said Sid, "I shut the top to check whether I could fit inside and now can't get the top open again – it would be ideal if you help to get me out."
Individually the creatures attempted to prise open the cover of the shell, yet it was stuck closed. "I can't perceive how we will get this top open," said Ears Mouse, "it's stuck shut." Simply then, he had a thought and murmured something in Alex's ear. Alex found a workable pace and hit the enormous shell with his foot. The shell top flew open, and Sid leaped out just in the event that it shut once more. "What did you murmur into Alex's car?" asked Molly. "I revealed to Alex that a goliath shell might have a monster carrot under it," giggled Ears Mouse.

Sid removed a carrot from his backpack and offered it to Alex to express gratitude toward him for liberating him from the monster shell.

Time was slipping away at this point, and everybody concurred that they would be advised to set home before it got dull. They got together their cover and excursion remains and put them into their backpacks. Alex set down and let them all trip onto his back, and they began their direction home.

In any case, they didn't get far before Alex stopped. "What's up, Alex?" asked Sid. "Nothing," said Alex, this is exactly what jackasses do now and again. "So, what would we be able to do to make your move once more?" asked Sid. "Have you got a carrot?" Alex inquired. When Sid revealed to him that he made them stay in his backpack, Alex guided him to tie it on the finish of a stick and to dangle it before Alex's nose. Sid severed a part of a hazel shrubbery and tied the carrot onto the finish of the branch with a pink lace that Molly leaned him. Much the same as enchantment, Alex began to walk again following the carrot before him.

It was not some time before they landed back at Alex's field, which Sid opened and shut as he had done previously. "Much appreciated Alex," they all yelled as they waved farewell to him. Sid gave Alex the last carrot, which he delighted in.

"Everybody returning to my place for some pleasant toast and Jim?" asked Ears Mouse. "Truly, please," they all said. They had truly made the most of their seaside adventure today.

That night Alex had a flawless dream about a mammoth carrot stowing away under a monster shell by the beach and nodded off with a major grin all over.

Have a good night rest.

2. The Swans and the Turtle

Sometimes ago,
There was a lake at the edges of a little town. Two swans and a turtle who were acceptable companions lived in the lake. They would play with one another and breathe easy recounting stories.

One year, there were no downpours, and the lake began evaporating.

"The lake is practically dry. We need to locate some other spot to live," said the turtle to the swans. "We will fly around and search for a reasonable spot," said the swans. Both the swans flew in various ways looking for a superior spot to live. A little separation away, one of the swans detected a huge lake. It had a lot of water, and there were numerous fishes in it. He flew back to tell the others.

Them three were extremely energized with the find. "Stunning! Presently we won't have any issue," said the turtle.

"There is just a single issue," answered one swan. "Both of us can fly there in a matter of moments. Be that as it may, you slither gradually. What's more, it is some separation away. You will never reach there."

The turtle thought for quite a while. Unexpectedly his face lit up. "I have a thought," he said. "You present to me a stick. I will hold the focal point of the stick in my mouth. Both of you can hold the stick on either side. That way, you can fly me with you to our new home."

"It is an awesome thought, yet you need to ensure you don't open your mouth in any way, shape, or form. On the off chance that you do, you will tumble to your demise," cautioned one of the swans.

The turtle concurred.

"Recollect what we let you know," reminded the swans as they prepared to fly. Before long, they were flying high in the sky. They needed to fly over the town to find a workable pace. As they flew over the town, individuals ran out into the streets to see this astonishing sight.

"What astute flying creatures. They are conveying a turtle on a stick!" shouted one man. Each one was eager to see such an astonishing sight.

"It was my thought. I am a shrewd one. I have to tell them," thought the turtle. He opened his mouth to clarify, yet before the absurd turtle could state anything, he fell with a crash and passed on.

The swans looked down at their dead companion and shook their heads sharply at his absurdity. "I he had kept his mouth shut, he would be alive and content with us," said one swan to the next as they arrived at the large lake, which would be their home from that point on.

3. The Three Little Pigs

A long time ago, when pigs could talk, and nobody had ever known about bacon, there experienced an old piggy mother with her three little children.

They had an exceptionally lovely home in an oak woodland, and were all similarly as upbeat as the day was long, until one miserable year the oak seed crop fizzled; at that point, undoubtedly, poor Mrs. Piggy-wiggy regularly had difficult work to make a decent living.

One day she called her children to her, and, with tears in her eyes, revealed to them that she should send them out into the wide world to look for their fortune.

She kissed them all round, and the three little pigs set out upon their movements, each taking an alternate street, and conveying a group threw on a stick over his shoulder.

The principal little pig had not gone far before he met a man conveying a heap of straw, so he said to him: "If it's not too much trouble, man, give me that straw to manufacture me a house?" The man was generally excellent natured, so he gave him the heap of straw, and the little pig constructed an entirely little house with it.

No sooner was it completed, and the little pig considering hitting the hay, than a wolf tagged along, thumped at the entryway, and stated: "Little pig, little pig, let me come in."

Be that as it may, the little pig giggled delicately, and replied: "No, no, by the hair of my chinny-jawline jaw."

At that point said the wolf harshly: "I will make you let me in, for I'll spat, and I'll puff, and I'll blow your home in.

He puffed, and he blew his home in, on the grounds that it was distinctly of straw and excessively light; and when he had blown the house in, he gobbled up the little pig, and didn't leave to such an extent as the tip of his tail.

The subsequent little pig likewise met a man, and he was conveying a heap of furze, so piggy said amiably: "It would be ideal if you kind man, will you give me that furze to manufacture me a house?"

The man concurred, and piggy set to work to fabricate himself a cozy little house before the night went ahead. It was hardly completed when the wolf went along and stated: "Little pig, little pig, let me come in."

"No, no, by the hair of my chinny-jawline jaw," addressed the subsequent little pig.

"At that point, I'll fit, and I'll puff, and I'll blow your home in!" said the wolf. He puffed severally, and finally, he blew the house in and ate the little pig up in a trice.

Presently, the third little pig met a man with a heap of blocks and mortar, and he stated: "Kindly man, will you give me those blocks to manufacture a house with?"

So the man gave him the blocks and mortar, and a little trowel also, and the little pig manufactured himself a decent solid little house. When it was done, the wolf came to call, similarly as he had done to the next little pigs, and stated: "Little pig, little pig, let me in!"

Be that as it may, the little pig replied: "No, no, by the hair of my chinny-jawline jaw."

"At that point," said the wolf, "I'll watch the episode, and I'll puff, and I'll blow your home in."

All things considered, he huffed, and he puffed, and he puffed, and he huffed, and he huffed, and he puffed; however, he couldn't get the house down. Finally, he had no breath left to the episode and puff with, so he plunked down outside the little pig's home and thought for momentarily.

Directly he got out: "Little pig, I know where there is a decent field of turnips."

"Where?" said the little pig.

"Behind the rancher's home, three fields away, and on the off chance that you will be prepared to-morrow morning, I will call for you, and we will go together and get some morning meal."

"Great," said the little Pig; "I will make certain to be prepared. What time do you intend to begin?"

"At six o'clock," answered the wolf.

All things considered, the savvy little pig found a good pace, hastened away to the field, and brought home a fine heap of turnips before the wolf came. At six o'clock, the wolf went to the little pig's home and stated: "Little pig, would you say you are prepared?"

"Prepared!" cried the little pig. "Why I have been to the field and return sometime in the past, and now I am occupied with heating up a potful of turnips for breakfast."

The wolf was exceptionally furious in fact; however, he decided to get the little pig in one way or another or other; so he revealed to him that he knew where there was a decent apple-tree.

"Where?" said the little pig.

"Round the slope in the squire's plantation," the wolf said. "So, on the off chance that you will vow to play me no stunts, I will want you tomorrow first thing at five o'clock, and we will go there together and get some ruddy-cheeked apples."

The following morning piggy found a good pace o'clock and was off and away sometime before the wolf came.

In any case, the plantation was far off; what's more, he had the tree to climb, which is a troublesome issue for a little pig, so that before the sack he had carried with him was very filled, he saw the wolf coming towards him.
He was appallingly scared. However, he thought it better to put a decent face on the issue, so when the wolf stated: "Little pig, what are you doing here before me? Are they decent apples?" he answered without a moment's delay: "Truly, very; I will toss down one for you to taste." So he picked an apple and tossed it so far that while the wolf was rushing to get it, he had the opportunity to bounce down and hurry away home.

The following day the wolf came back once more, and told the little pig that there would have been reasonable in the town that evening, and inquired as to whether he would go with him.

"Goodness! Indeed," said the pig, "I will go with joy. What time will you be prepared to begin?"

"At half-past three," said the wolf.

Obviously, the little pig began well before the time, went to the reasonable, and purchased a fine enormous margarine beat, and was running endlessly with it on his back when he saw the wolf coming.

He didn't have the idea what to do, so he crawled into the beat to stow away, and by so doing began it rolling.

Down the slope, it went, turning again and again, with the little pig squeaking inside.

The wolf couldn't think what the abnormal thing moving down the slope could be, so he retreated in a fear home in dread while never set off to the reasonable. He went to the little pig's home to disclose to him how scared he had been by a huge round thing which came moving past him down the slope.

"Ha! ha!" giggled the little pig, "so I scared you, eh? I had been to the reasonable and purchased margarine agitate; when I saw you, I got inside it and moved down the slope."

This exasperated the wolf that he pronounced that he would gobble up the little pig and that nothing should spare him, for he would hop down the stack.

Be that as it may, the smart little pig hung a pot loaded with water over the hearth and afterward made a bursting fire, and similarly, as the wolf was descending the stack, he removed the spread and in fell the wolf. In a second, the little pig had popped the top on once more.

At that point, he heated up the wolf and ate him for dinner, and after that, he lived unobtrusively and serenely the entirety of his days and was never upset by a wolf again.

4. The Cat and The Mouse in Partnership

A CAT having made the associate of a mouse, advised her such an extensive amount the incredible love and love that he had for her, that the mouse finally agreed to live in a similar house with him and to share their household undertakings for all intents and purpose. "Yet, we should accommodate the winter," said the feline, "or we will be famished; you, little mouse, can't go wherever searching for nourishment, or you will meet with a mishap."

This counsel was followed, and a pot was carried with some oil in it. Be that as it may, when they had got it, they couldn't envision where it ought to be put; however finally, after a long thought, the feline stated: "I realize no preferred spot to put it over in the congregation, for there nobody sets out to take anything; we will set it underneath the organ, and not contact it till we truly need it."

So the pot was taken care of in wellbeing, yet not long a while later the feline started to want for it once more, so he addressed the mouse and stated: "I need to reveal to you that I am asked by my auntie to stand adoptive parent to a little child, white with dark-colored imprints, whom she has recently brought into the world. Thus I should go to the initiating. Release me out today, and do you stop at home and keep the house."

"Surely," addressed the mouse, "implore, go, and in the event that you eat anything decent, consider me; I would likewise enthusiastically drink a tad bit of the sweet red dedicating wine."

Be that as it may, oh! It was each of them a story; for the feline had no auntie, and had not been approached to stand back up the parent to anyone. He went directly to the congregation, crawled up to the oil pot, and licked it till he had eaten off the top; at that point he went for a stroll on the tops of the houses in the town, thoroughly considering his circumstance, and from time to time extending himself in the sun and stroking his hairs as frequently as he suspected of his supper. At the point when it was evening, he returned home once more, and the mouse stated: "So you have come finally; what an enchanting day you more likely than not had!"

"Truly," addressed the feline; "it went off well overall!"

"What have you named the little cat?" asked the mouse.

"Top-off," said the feline rapidly.

"Top-off!" answered the mouse; "that is an inquisitive and striking name; is it normal in your family?"

"What does that make a difference?" said the feline; "it isn't more terrible than Crumb-stealer, as your kids are called."

Not long subsequently the feline felt a similar aching as in the past, and said to the mouse: "You should oblige me by dealing with the house again independent from anyone else; I am again approached to stand adoptive parent, and, since the youth has a white ring round his neck, I can't get off the greeting." So the great little mouse agreed, and the feline crawled away behind the divider to the congregation once more and ate a large portion of the substance of the oil pot. "Nothing tastes superior to anything that one eats by one's self," said he, very placated with his day's worth of effort, and when he got back home, the mouse asked how this kid was named.

"Half-out," addressed the feline.

"Half-out! I don't get your meaning? I will bet anything it isn't in the schedule," yet the feline answered nothing.

Pussy's mouth before long started to water again at the memory of the devouring. "Every beneficial thing comes in threes," said he to the mouse. "I am again required to be back up parent; this kid is very dark, and has minimal white paws, however not a solitary white hair on his body; a wonder such as this just happens once in two years, so supplicate pardon me this time."

"Top-off! Half-out!" addressed the mouse; "those are such inquisitive names, they make me somewhat suspicious."

"Ok!" answered the feline, "there you sit in your dim cover and long tail, thinking drivel. That happens to fail to go out."

The mouse busied herself during the feline's nonappearance in taking care of the house. However, in the interim insatiable puss licked the oil pot clear out. "At the point when it is altogether done, one will find happiness in the hereafter," thought he to himself, and when night came, he returned home fat and tired. The mouse, in any case, again asked what name the third kid had gotten. "It won't satisfy you any better," addressed the feline, "for he is gotten All-out."

"Full scale!" shouted the mouse; "well, that is unquestionably the most inquisitive name by a long shot. I have never yet observed it in print. Hard and fast! What would that be able to mean?" and, shaking her head, she moved up and rested.

After that no one else requested that the feline stand back up parent; yet the winter had shown up, and nothing more was to be selected up from entryways; so the mouse bethought herself of their store of arrangement, and stated, "Come, companion feline, we will go to our oil pot which we laid by; it will taste well at this point."

"Truly, in fact," answered the feline; "it will taste just as on the off chance that you stroked your tongue against the window."

So they set out on their adventure, and when they landed at the congregation, the pot remained in its old spot—yet it was unfilled! "Ok," said the mouse, "I see what has occurred; presently, I realize you are to be sure a devoted companion. You have eaten the entire as you stood guardian; first Top-off, at that point Half-out, at that point—"

"Will you hush up?" cried the feline. "Not a word, or I'll eat you." But the poor mouse had "Hard and fast" at her tongue's end, and had barely expressed it when the feline made a spring, held onto her in his mouth, and gulped her.

This happens each day on the planet.

5. Tropical Adventure in the Magic Shed

Quite a long time ago, One splendid sunny day, Molly went to Sophie's home for a Sunday play date. "What are we going to play today?" Molly inquired. "What about football? It is the World Cup nowadays!" And with that, they joyfully jumped to the back yard. They were making some dazzling memories until the ball hit the enchantment shed. Right then and there, Sophie felt a shiver of energy. "We haven't been in the shed for quite a while!" Dearest perusers, Molly and Sophie, have had numerous adventures in the enchanted shed, yet they had checked a few times and hadn't found any mystical signs during the previous scarcely any weeks.

Molly hurried to the freeboard yet slipped on a thick green leaf. Molly and Sophie went into the passage when unexpectedly, Sophie said, "The passage is getting increasingly damp, and tropical leaves are going ahead of my face. We are presumably heading off to a tropical rainforest!" She had speculated accurately as they passed a wooden sign denoted 'The Amazon rainforest' and entered the tropical land. "Molly!" shouted Sophie, "that is no joke!" Just at that point, Molly detected a lake close by and took a gander at her appearance and saw a major fierceness body with dark stripes and two feline ears roosted on her head!

A couple of moments later, they heard strides moving ever closer. Molly and Sophie covered up in a major shrubbery near a fix of trees. The strides had a place with lumberjacks. A tiny bit at a time, they viewed the men chop down the lovely trees. After the men left, Sophie asked Molly, "Do you believe we're here to stop deforestation?" Molly gestured worriedly. "So first we have to

caution the creatures… and you ought to do it" completed Sophie, and with that, Molly made an uproarious "ROAR!" "I will follow the men and discover what they're doing and what their identity is," Sophie told Molly and ran into the trees.
After a couple of seconds, directly before Molly were furious tigers, bright toucans, brilliant frogs, and uncommon pink dolphins in a stream close by. "Are you OK?" Asked a pink dolphin. "Truly yet, I saw a few men come and cut an excellent piece of the woodland. Do you know what their identity is?" asked Molly. "They are lumberjacks, individuals whose activity is to chop down trees!" Exclaimed a gold frog. "Also, on the off chance that they keep this up, we'll have nowhere to live!" Added a tiger.

Sophie was unobtrusively following the men until they halted before a colossal tent. Beside the tent, there was an enormous seat with a mean, thin man on it, and he said, "Dubai requested 200kg of wood, and you brought 100kg to bring 100kg by sunset, or something bad might happen… " Sophie hurried into the woodland and said to the men, "You need to quit chopping down trees, it's stinging the creatures that live here!" "Move over, young lady! We just take orders from our chief." After that, they moved to the following gathering of trees. Sophie raced to Molly and disclosed to her that the lumberjacks weren't tuning in. Molly informed Sophie concerning an arrangement that the creatures were going to encompass the lumberjacks, then Sophie could converse with them, and that is actually what they did. At the point when the lumberjacks looked to one side, there was a fix of trees with furious toucans prepared to peck. At the point when they looked on their right side, there were snarling tigers! What's more, when they thought of hopping into the waterway behind them, there were pink dolphins splashing them from head to toe, lastly Sophie before them. Out of nowhere, Sophie said, "Amazon rainforest is ensured. What you're doing is illicit, and in the event that you don't stop, I'll report you to the police, however, I won't call them in the event that you assist us with calling the Dubai organization and mention to them what's happening," completed Sophie. A few lumberjacks were persuaded and promptly took out their telephones and told the organization that the trees they are getting are from the Amazon Rainforest. Sophie had an extraordinary thought and took the telephone from one of the lumberjacks and gave the organization making the greatest nursery in the entire world, as of now, has the world's tallest structure and greatest shopping center. The organization promptly concurred on the grounds that they cherished greenery in the desert, and the lumberjacks' supervisor went to prison.

The creatures were thankful and arranged a gathering with a tropical organic product like mangoes, mythical serpent natural products, durian, pineapples, and bananas and loads of orchid flowers. A tiger gave Sophie and Molly a brilliant seed to plant at their home as a present. "At the point when it's a tree, it will have gold leaves," he said. Sophie and Molly cheerfully said thank you and farewell. They experienced the passage and plunked down on their bed for a very much earned rest. The following day, they painstakingly planted their seeds and thought of their Rainforest Adventure.

6. The Adventures of Sprinkles The Cat; The King

Quite a long time ago, Imagine maybe, a realm based upon a distant shore. A realm where the streets were fixed with valuable pearls that dispersed the sunlight onto the entirety of the houses inside its fringes. The waters are running delicately into the cliffside, just as the two were moving.

The most wonderful spot is possible. The realm of Nepeta Cataria, home of felines. This is the place our story happens.

Ruler Tom managed the land with an iron clench hand. He was a brutal and wild lord who thought more about realms' excellence than the individuals who lived inside its fringes. He was set to guarantee all grounds close and far, without the slightest hesitation of the lives, he might be placed at serious risk.

His military was the biggest in cat history; however, at last, they were no counterpart for the sort hearted warrior referred to over the grounds as Sprinkles the feline. With his quieting murmur and his caring look, he could make even the most devoted fighters leave in harmony. Moms never again cried in the streets, hanging tight for the protected return of their youngsters. Wherever he went, he carried harmony and quietness with him. He was genuinely a related soul, shrewd past his years.

One night as the lord plunked down for his supper, he heard the news that a feline had gotten more broadly known and regarded than him, and this irritated him. "I request that you catch this feline and toss him in the cell! Who does he think he is? This is my territory!" Said the ruler.

So the troopers were conveyed with another strategy. To catch Sprinkles, in any condition. Following quite a while of preparing, they were sure they could do it. However, as each troop of men went out, they stayed away forever. As this proceeded, the ruler just got increasingly enraged. His kin was drained, eager, injured. They lived in dread of Sprinkles, as their friends and family left and stayed away forever home. They were losing any expectation of consistently observing them once more.

At that point on one steadfast day, felines were seen walking upon the skyline towards the realm. An extraordinary feline, the entirety of the missing troopers. Be that as it may, they never again spread a message of viciousness. They gained from Sprinkles the methods for graciousness and liberality. What's more, they had set out, spreading the message to all that would tune in. As they spilled out into the streets and were brought together with their families, the realm celebrated. Their whimpers could be gotten notification from miles away as they embraced and licked one another. Children and fathers together once more.

Everybody was cheerful — all things considered, nearly everybody. The ruler was distraught. His arrangements had all been thwarted. Hearts as dark and cold as he would set aside some effort to fix. His own troopers broke into his castle, pulled him from his honored position, and tossed him in prison. Capital punishment was run of the mill under his rule. However, his destiny was still in question.

The realm cast a ballot that the crown ought to go to Sprinkles The Cat, their guardian angel, and now their ruler. As he developed more established, he wedded and had little cats. He showed them, alongside the realm, that consideration consistently wins. He said, "Let it be realized that in any event, when a fight is lost, and material things are gone, the benevolence in an individual's heart is the most important fortune of all."

With respect to the previous lord, he invested energy in prison, yet was in the long run discharged depending on the prerequisite that he be declawed and go to a multi-week outrage the board course followed by treatment for an incredible length.

The End

7. A Queer Friendship

Max pooch and Lucy crow were the best of companions. Be that as it may, theirs was an abnormal fellowship since Max was hard of hearing, and Lucy was weak. Having harmed her left-wing and leg, which had been squashed under the wheels of a vehicle, Lucy couldn't fly. In this way, the entire day, she sat roosted on Max's back, and the canine conveyed her to places where nourishment was accessible, similar to the side of the road dustbins and parks.

The two companions were cheerful in one another's organization and cherished and regarded one another.

Different creatures, in the area, additionally valued this strange fellowship and constantly supported it. Be that as it may, fiasco struck one day, with the approach of the rainstorm. The whole zone was overflowed. Subsequently, men and cows kicked the bucket, and houses were assaulted, and vegetation was obliterated. Debilitated and cold, Lucy and Max chose to leave the region and move to another spot. Conveying Lucy on his back, Max walked along the street, halting just around evening time to rest.

In the long run, they went to another town, where the individuals were rich, and dustbins and side of the road were constantly covered with nourishment. Max and Lucy chose to remain and make it their new home. They were cheerful, yet the others were definitely not. They got envious of the two companions. Leo, a street hound, considered Max an imbecile and stated, "You are an inept insane canine." Why else would you convey that faltering crow on your back? What utilize would that pointless winged creature be to you?" Chinni sparrow considered Lucy a parasite and reproached her for exploiting a poor hard of hearing canine. The crows of the area didn't converse with Lucy since, rather than their organization, she liked to be agreeable with Max. As far as concerns them, the street hounds kept away from Max, since he had brought down himself by keeping organization with a typical crow.

Hearing this, Max just snickered, yet Lucy got pitiful. "I am futile," she thought. "I have consistently let Max thoroughly take care of me. However, I have never done anything for him, nor helped him in any capacity". As days passed, Lucy turned out to be increasingly tragic. "I should accomplish something for Max, to give him that I cherish and value his kinship a ton."

At some point, it was evening, and Max was resting on one roadside. Lucy, who was sitting close to Max, out of nowhere, detected a huge meat bone that had fallen on the ground, from the butcher's shop on the contrary roadside. Her eyes illuminated. "Let me get that bit of bone for Max. Thinking thus, she limped over the street, hauling her left leg. Twisting, she got the bit of bone, with her Ray and was going across the street, when she saw a vehicle coming at max throttle, serving to one side and right. She likewise observed that Max had turned over in his rest and was currently extended most of the way over the street. "I should caution him." Lucy froze and thought. Following up hastily, Lucy tossed the bone energetically at Max. Frightened, Max opened his eyes and saw the vehicle. Acting in a flash, he bounced across to wellbeing.

Lucy had spared Max's life, every one of the creatures and fowls presently began regarding Lucy.

8. Dinosaurs In My Bed

Andrew lay shuddering in his bed. The sky was bursting at the seams with blasting sounds and splendid flashes simply outside his window.

Fifteen minutes back, he asked, "Mother, will the tempest keep going long?"

"Kindly, don't stress," she said. "The meteorologist guaranteed it would ignore Truro rapidly. Presently get some rest."

But it didn't, and he proved unable.

Andrew tuned in to his morning timer. "Tick... Tick... Tock." The night appeared to go on until the end of time. Seconds transformed into minutes.

At that point, into what appeared hours.

Over the house, noisy lightning crashes made him duck further under the covers. Outside thunder even shook his window.

Would it be a good idea for him to go into his parent's room? If, he was a major kid now. What's more, he must be daring. Father even helped him get ready for this awful climate.
Just on the off chance that it endured throughout the night.

Presently his knapsack was covered up under the covers. It was loaded up with most loved toys, games, and comic books. Indeed "Panda" bear he had since the age of two.

The mother ensured Andrew additionally had a couple of treats. A gigantic pack of popcorn was near his correct side. What's more, a pack of undulated chips was on the other.

His family had gone rising in Cape Breton, a weekend ago. So he was currently a kid with outdoor understanding. Also, he realized how he would generally be courageous.

What was moving around his toes? "Ouch, that hurt," his trembling voice, murmured. The commotion outside was so boisterous Andrew could barely think.

Through the window, a dull sky shut out the stars.

The kid was out of nowhere, anxious. What was under the cover? He was interested and scrounged through his rucksack.

"OMIGOSH," Andrew said. "I overlooked my spotlight."

He slid up and flung himself over the floor. Andrew chased around until he discovered it in the top closet space.

Rapidly hopping go into bed, he constrained cold feet down to the end. Uncovered toes laid on something harsh and sharp. Presently it was by all accounts slithering around his lower legs.

Wow! He wasn't the only one in bed!

He checked under the spreads where it was dark as coal, practically like being outside. Rather than shining stars lit up, spots looked increasingly like eyes.

Thundering originated from behind his left leg.

Andrew bit to his left side thumb and turned on the spotlight. "That unnerving sound couldn't be… ?" he delayed.

Truly, a dinosaur! Be that as it may, that was unimaginable, would it say it wasn't? Dinosaurs couldn't fit under bed blankets, having a place with a young man, living inside his home. Isn't that so?

Wrong. Gazing back at him was a Stegosaurus. What's more, it tasted his Hostess vinegar chips, the one little sack with a couple of pieces left.

"Escape, you!" Andrew roared, attempting to be bold. The creature thundered something back under the sweeping sky and rushed into a shadowy corner.

New commotions got the kid's consideration. His electric lamp helped choose moving shadows. What was happening? He pondered. There was a Triceratops and a Deinonychus.

Also, a Tyrannosaurus!

"Run!" Andrew shouted. Out of nowhere, he had a feeling that he was just a single alive on the planet. In any case, he was still under his cover that appeared to grow out yonder and even high above him.

He scanned for someplace to stow away.

Cold feet could scarcely move. It resembled an alternate world under the covers. His heart walked to the beat of a drum. Lightning zipped, then destroyed under his sweeping sky.

Huge creatures started to pursue littler ones.

Dashing toward him was a Dicraeosaurus. This was a quiet plant-eater and would not hurt him. In any case, Andrew couldn't take any risks.

He pulled a fire motor from his knapsack. Bouncing into the front seat, Andrew turned the alarm on full speed. Everything it did was harmed his ears.

A Ceratosaurus and Albertosaurus limited after him. They resembled enormous neighborly pooches needing to play. Be that as it may, Andrew didn't wish to get squashed.

He hurried up pedal. Furthermore, the firing motor jumped forward.

Before long, the street turned into a restricted way, pointing straight for the woods. Andrew immediately stopped. At that point, he bound on new tennis shoes from his knapsack.

He likewise brought his whistle. High pitched blowing cautioned everything to escape his direction. A whirlwind of feet got away down the path, each progression beating hard.

One arm held firmly to 'Panda.'

The breeze passed over his top, sending it into the separation. Branches grabbed at his face. He would not like to get squashed or eaten by those dinosaurs.

The tempest outside was nothing contrasted with wild creatures pursuing him under his cover. How did the entirety of this occur in any case?

Snarls and speeding feet kept pace behind him. Venturing into his rucksack, Andrew snatched his in-line skates. Presently, he figured, it ought to be anything but difficult to skate away securely.

That is until a subtle tree root sent him carelessly into the mud.

Presently it was pick up the pace time to climb a tree.

"Mother, where are you?" Andrew yelled. "Daddy!" Skinny legs mixed up the storage compartment. What's more, similar to a monkey moved higher from branch to branch.

Out of nowhere between two appendages was the leader of a Brontosaurus. It grinned as it bit a significant piece of leaves. "What's your concern?" it appeared to state.

"Andrew! ANDREWWW!" somebody called. Voices appeared to move to and fro and around like echoes. Truly, individuals were yelling his name!

The kid hurriedly lost his covers, sat up, and gazed at mother and father. He flickered as morning's sun looked between Venetian blinds.

"Panda" was as yet tucked safely under his arm.

"I see you found our shocks under your covers," mother said.

Andrew took a gander at his mother.

"You know. Recollect the dinosaur models you requested a week ago?"

"What's more, I'm glad for you," father said. "Look how perfectly you stacked them on your wardrobe."

Andrew felt peculiar as his father pointed.

In a perfect line was a procession of brilliant dinosaurs. They were following a benevolent Dicraeosaurus, with a fierce-looking Tyrannosaurus Rex toward the stopping point.

Driving the entire gathering was a figure of a young man.

Also, he was holding firmly to a teddy bear.

9. Ginger and the six felines

Some time ago

It was a dazzling day in the glade, and the entirety of ginger's six siblings and sisters were playing in the knoll's naturally developed grass.

Every last bit of her siblings and sisters were dim, yet ginger was a gold shading with orange stripes. Gingers sibling's and sister's names were; Gray, Tom, Linx, Victoria, Petunia, and Polly. Ginger's siblings and sisters prodded her since she had ginger shaded hide, and they all had dark-hued hide. This made ginger tragic. For the most part, on days like this present, ginger's siblings and sisters wouldn't allow her to play. So ginger would sit underneath a tree in the shade while she watched her siblings and sisters play in the lovely warm knoll.

A couple of days after the fact, the news spread that the feline races were going to start in 3 days. Ginger and her siblings and sisters murmured up. The entirety of ginger's siblings and sisters were amazed that ginger pursued the feline races. "Why'd ginger sign up?" Victoria murmured to Polly. "Better believe it," concurred Tom. "Ginger's such a major fraidy-feline. She'll likely be frightened to such an extent that she won't have the option to move. At that point, I'll zoom directly past her and be the first to the end goal," said Linx. "What are you TALKING about?!" whimpered Petunia. "Don't you mean I'll be first to the end goal?" "Don't you mean I will?" As ginger's siblings and sisters kept on arguing, ginger arranged for the enormous race. She was timing herself as she did laps around the knoll.

On a large day, she was prepared. Dim, Tom, Petunia, Linx, Polly Victoria, and ginger were altogether arranged at the beginning line at the Claw-vill dashing foundation. The cougar ref was standing by persistently to drop the banner.

While ginger and her siblings are sisters were trusting that the banner will drop, gingerly pulled out the guide to see where the course went. At the present time, they were at the passageway of the Claw-vill shopping center.

The race was from the earliest starting point of the shopping center right to the finish of the shopping center. The shopping center was extremely mainstream, so it was, in every case, exceptionally occupied. Since the shopping center was so occupied, it got extended to a length of 1 MILE LONG.

At the point when ginger set away from her guide, there was just a single additional MINUTE until the banner dropped. So one moment later, the banner dropped. The race had BEGUN!

Linx, the quickest of the litter, was in the number one spot. Ginger was following behind. At that point, different young men got up to speed with Linx. "Hello, Linx!" gasped Tom. "Since different young ladies are so moderate, we should 'stop at the salmon shack to get some food?" "OK," said Linx, not exhausted.

In the meantime, ginger and her sisters were still in the race. With Ginger still behind, Petunia was leading the pack. Polly and Victoria got up to speed with her. "Hello! Wanna stop at the 'pretty kitty' hide salon? It's right up ahead." "Alright, sure. Ginger should, in any case, be behind when we're set."

So now, just ginger was in the race. She was hoping to land toward the end goal and see Linx wearing an in front of the rest of the competition decoration and every last bit of her different siblings and sisters WAILING since they didn't WIN. What's more, When ginger FINALLY landed toward the end goal, her jaw dropped. None of her siblings or sisters were there! No. This couldn't be correct. Perhaps they all returned to the lair since she was taking to long.

In any case, when the puma saw Ginger toward the end goal, she said enthusiastically, "Congrats! You simply WON the Claw-vill feline race!" Ginger got gave a blessing crate with a major brilliant jar of sardines and a purple wad of yarn within it. Ginger could barely handle it. She had quite recently WON the greatest race of the year!

Ginger returned home with her presents and calculated that her siblings and sisters would return home once they understood what had occurred. At the point when her siblings and sisters returned home, they were all wailing since they didn't win and in light of the fact that they were heartbroken. "We're all so grieved, Ginger." Said Petunia over her tears. At that point, they gave Ginger a major embrace. After that, Ginger pardoned them and gave them each a sardine from her brilliant can. What's more, from that point onward, they all lived cheerfully ever after.

10. Kyle the Monkey

At some point, a gathering of four companions chose to visit the nearby jubilee, which had halted in the town for the end of the week. It just came once per year, and the gathering of companions was quick to investigate the miracle of the Jimboree. The sounds and the sights were so energizing, and among delightful fields, it made for an exceptional occasion. Rose, Samantha, Vanessa, and Jimes were as glad as anybody that this end of the week had at last shown up. They carried their pet monkey alongside them to partake in the good times. His name was Kyle, and with the gentlest grin and amazing eyes, a lot of the locals had a fondness for Kyle. The individuals who ran the Jimboree originated from various nations and communicated in various dialects. Kyle had never gone to a jubilee, and his proprietors were sharp.
Upon landing in the festival, the gathering of four companions got in near discussion about where they should head first. They immediately made up their psyches to set out toward the spooky house and turned around to take Kyle with them. Incredibly, Kyle was not there. He had vanished among the groups, causing frenzy and stress among the four companions.

"Dread not!" yelled Rose, "We will utilize our abilities among this festival society to locate our darling, Kyle." Every one of the four companions had an expertise that was useful in discovering lost individuals or creatures; they had done it before to locate Samantha's more youthful sister, Rachel. Rose could do a drawing of who was missing with the goal that she could inquire as to whether they had seen anybody looking like Kyle. Samantha communicated in numerous dialects and could ask any individuals from another nation on the off chance that they had seen Kyle. Vanessa had the option to do the sounds and activities of Kyle to check whether anybody remembered them, and Jimes could ask and request in melody with respect to whether anybody had seen his dearest, Kyle.

They attempted to discover Kyle at the Haunted House, where a man was taking care of the ride. Rose drew an image of Kyle and inquired:

"Have you seen my Kyle?"

The man snorted, and it appeared he didn't know English. Samantha immediately asked the man in another dialect on the off chance that he knew where Kyle was. The man replied so that each of the four of the companions realized that Kyle was not at the Haunted House.

Next, they went to the teacups, where Vanessa did the sounds and activities that Kyle typically does. The lady caring for the teacups snickered and dismissed. Jimes started to sing and utilized his tune to pose an inquiry, and the lady considered this, and answered: "I'm sorry, my dear, I have not seen your monkey."

At long last, they went to the merry go round, trusting that Kyle would be there someplace. Rose gave her attracting of Kyle to individuals, yet no one knew where Kyle was. Jimes sang. However, no one replied back. Samantha posed inquiries in numerous dialects, yet nothing worth mentioning news came. At long last, Vanessa did the sounds that Kyle makes, and comparable sounds originated from the merry go round. Kyle ran towards the four companions, who grasped Kyle for what felt like an unfathomable length of time. The four companions and Kyle clasped hands for the remainder of the day, so they would not lose each other until the end of time. They went on every one of the rides until the sun went down, and left the Jimboree that night, anticipating its arrival one year from now.

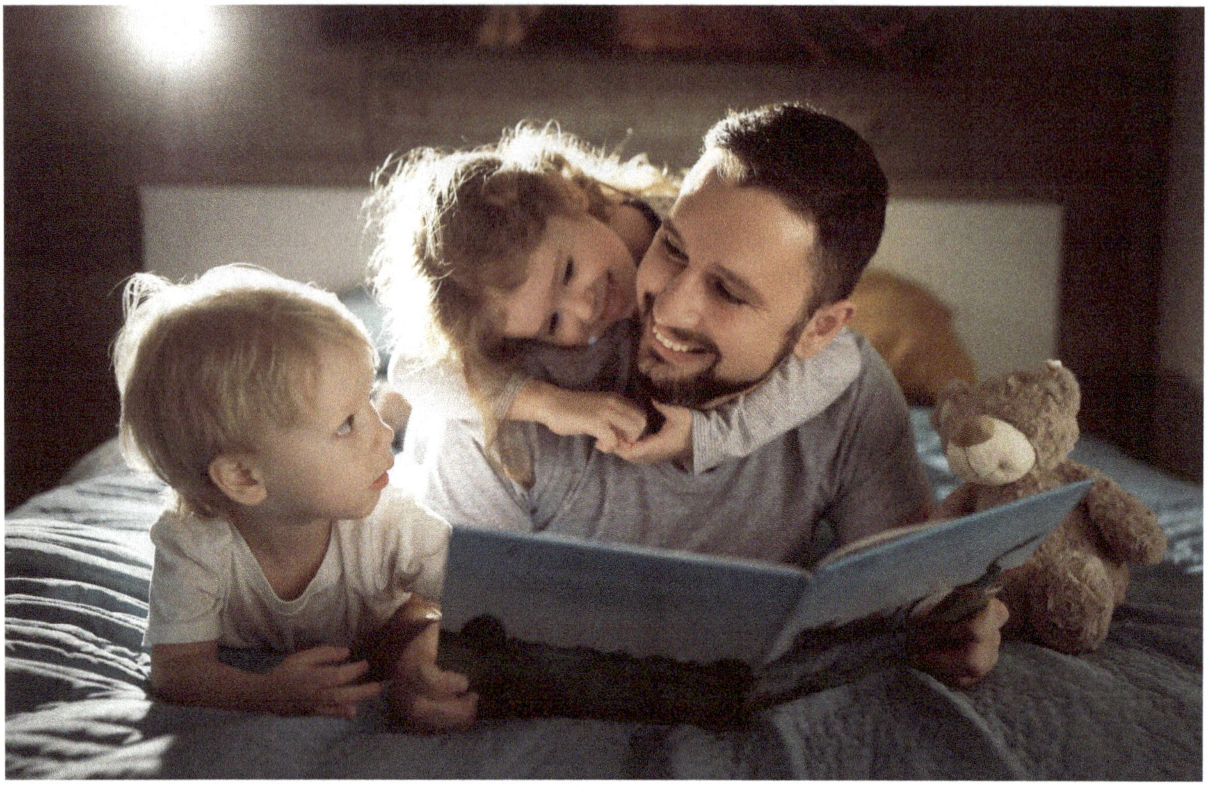